STOP PROCRASTINATING

A Strategic Program To Increase Productivity, Overcome Procrastination, Build Self-Discipline And Start Living

By

Peter Harding

The information herein is offered for informational purposes solely and is universal as so. The presentation of the information is without contract or any type of guarantee assurance.

The trademarks that are used are without any consent, and the publication of the trademark is without permission or backing by the trademark owner. All trademarks and brands within this book are for clarifying purposes only and are the owned by the owners themselves, not affiliated with this document.

Page intentionally left blank

TABLE OF CONTENTS

INTRODUCTION

Procrastination is the practice of putting an action or duty off or stopping it until later. This term comes from the Latin "pro," which means "in, forward or for" and "crastinus," which means "for tomorrow."

Many find Procrastination to be a negative, counterproductive behavior. Nevertheless, it is rarely seen in a positive light. It was pointed out by some writers as a practical pause or as avoiding hurry. Nevertheless, as demonstrated in the subsequent historical study, the positive form of procrastination is only secondary in usage.

This GUIDE focuses on the most negative aspect of procrastinations. Like the other common terms described in the scientific study, definitions of procrastination are almost as extensive as the people who study this topic. At first, such a shift in meaning can seem to confuse the essence of procrastination, but in certain respects can be used to illuminate it partially.

Most researchers' attempts to refine their interpretation of meaning are more compatible than contradictory. In addition, every common concept only shows a central or necessary element.

It is apparent that all meanings and conceptualizations of procrastination suggest that a task or decision must be deferred, procrastinated or put off in line with the Latin root of the term.

A procrastinator is, on that basis, anyone who puts off the start or completion of an event or mission. That distinction is significant, as there are hundreds of tasks you can do at any time and it is difficult to think that you put them off.

Procrastination is especially widespread nowadays. It seems like everybody is afflicted with it. It's like a modern disease which knows no race, sex, age or limit. Some of us may have put off things from time to time, but it's a way of life for others.

Why are so many people procrastinating? Have we been raised like this? I think that the answer is a major NO. We're becoming conditioned repellents. One of the reasons is that we do not see what causes procrastination. Many who try to avoid procrastination first have to identify the root causes and when you know why you will make improvements to solve procrastinations.

Fortunately, there have been specific physiological analysis on procrastination, and, after all, major reasons that lead to it. We shall look in-depth into this topic and also devise a strategic program to increase productivity, overcome procrastination, build self-discipline and start living.

Are you ready?

Let's get started

CHAPTER 1
WHAT IS PROCRASTINATION?

For many people, procrastination is something with which they are too easily associated and identified. The challenge is that once you identify with a behavior (positive and negative) it becomes a part of who you are and that this identity filters your experiences and actions.

We may describe "work aversion" as the unreasonable procrastination of the expected course of action. Translated from the original Latin language, literally, the phrase 'for tomorrow' means procrastination. As human beings we still look for opportunities to be better off-and this we do with a good purpose.

Although procrastination seems to contradict this fact, it does indeed illustrate a very important point. This is not necessarily the result of the deliberate actions that we do, or fail to do, but also the result of causes that we do not realize consciously. When you do not take the action, you assume, on some level of your unconscious thought, that you would do worse if you take the action.

You have to do two things to change this negative tendency. First of all, you need to remove the association and 'attachments' that you could have with procrastination if you don't know you're a procrastinator.

Although you can often procrastinate, by identifying your actions you cannot afford to restrict yourself. Furthermore, you need to redefine procrastination so that it motivates and empowers you rather than limits you.

The way we describe things for ourselves defines how we communicate. If you see the latter as a chronic problem with which you have been born, you will probably struggle with it all your life. If you define procrastination as a bad habit that you will have to face somewhere in the future, it will control you. If you see the pause as something that you cannot solve, you'll probably be right.

When you describe procrastination as a negative propensity to set things aside, then through discontinuing it you will be motivated to act. The result of your ability is seldom whether you can do anything.

It's almost always a motivation case. Motivation is nothing but an inner drive which forces you to act, and it is a mighty thing to find the required motivation to make use of your abilities.

There is a description of procrastination that can do just that. I choose to define it as the time thief. You can see how real it is when you think about it because the uncertainty is what holds you immobilized and inactive.

Time is the most precious and useful commodity. People go to drastic measures to secure their money and properties, but don't "shield" their time – one thing that money can never buy.

Understanding to value your time is an effective tactic to tackle obstacles and make the most of your life. When you love something, you take care of it and defend it.

Your time is limited. Do you ever wonder how many days you've had in your life?

At first glance you might think it's 100,000 or even a million. In fact, your lifespan would be only 25,550 days if you grow to be 70 years old. If you are thirty now, then you have only another 260,000 hours left-and a third of that will go to sleep.

You have as much time on this planet as Mother Theresa, Bill Gates, Steve Jobs, Oprah Winfrey or anyone else. The only difference is how you spend your time. Don't allow your most precious possessions to be stolen.

Rather, see procrastination as a call to action. It is possible that what you're doing is something you 'must' do. See, what governs us what we do not do, and what we do not see. Yet when you face it and do it, you get free and it doesn't affect you anymore.

You don't allow the time thief to hold you when you have this sense of urgency and consciousness that your time is precious. What you get out of yourself is not dependent on your ability. It depends on how much of your money you can control and that is almost entirely an exercise in psychology. You will begin to shift this inner dialogue by changing how you perceive procrastination and allow yourself to act and make things happen.

We have been there. You were given 30 days to prepare a term paper, but did not start the paper until the day before its due date. This is called Procrastination. A wise man described procrastination as a "dream killer", because it destroys productivity. It is best to describe it as postponing, or postponed action to a later date. We all procrastinate now and then. It is an issue only if it stops or prevents us from living a complete and vibrant life.

Some of us work with administration tasks, some of us at home with homework, but one thing is clear, it can't be good for us or for people around us.

Are you aware that surveys have shown that approximately 20 percent of people consider themselves as, for example, buggers: for not being able to pay their bills on time; skipping job or promotion possibilities; no parking fees on time or saving their Christmas or birthday gift shopping until the last minute?

The reality is that procrastinators can put off doing things indefinitely – have you heard anyone say "I am going on a diet tomorrow"

There are many ways to interrupt our lives, but I agree that procrastination is one of the worst ways, after all, who wants a life of regret by not acting on time?

Generally speaking, we learn to Procrastinate and are not born with it. The procrastination of our parents, siblings or other authority figures may be observed when we grow up. It is sometimes an answer to a parenting authoritarian style. Controlling parents may discourage children from having the capacity to respond quickly without obtaining additional guidance from an official in their lives. Once we are adults, we can still try this additional guidance before acting, but at this stage the figures of authority may not be present, causing us to procrastinate. In some instances, procrastination may be a form of resistance or a way of being simply recognized. Procrastinators may turn to friends rather than families for help, but sadly our friends may exacerbate the problem by accepting our excuses.

There are many consequences of procrastination, for example, wellbeing. Studies show that procrastination can lead to more colds and flu, gastrointestinal issues and insomnia in the compromised immune systems. It can also remove responsibility from us and others, leading to resentment and destruction of teamwork and relations.

There are various types of procrastinators:

1. Those who leave tasks until the last minute and receive a buzz from frenzied last-minute activities – particularly when they have no choice.

2. Many with fear of failure – will also fear performance, but this fear prevents them from behaving either way. They can be very self-aware and worry about what others think of them.

3. Those that just want to stop decision taking. They take no responsibility for the outcome in this way.

There are a few strategies available to get rid of Procrastination from your life.

Through a lot of concentrated work, procrastinators are able to conquer their self-control. It takes a great deal of mental strength and can be very exhausting. Fortunately, however, there is a simple and efficient solution and it is found in the fields of NLP or Neuro-Linguistic Programming.

Cognitive therapies that help you think, and any difficulty you face will often do more harm than good. It doesn't mean they don't work, but other strategies like:

1. Anchoring- change the "trigger" effects, which usually cause you to replenish.

2. Change of behavior- break the behavior pattern before it manifests

3. Value alignment- discovery of values and beliefs that can lead to reproduction.

4. Integration of parts- removal of conflicting psyche parts

5. Negative emotion and removal of belief

These strategies are found so much quicker in the field of NLP than any other cognitive therapies and are almost instantly successful.

Whenever we practice procrastinations, it ultimately ruins our productivity – it kills our dreams. Just think for a minute: what would you do (that's worth doing) if you didn't take action? If you put off cleaning your house, you'll eventually live in a pig trap, not to mention health problems caused by maintenance problems.

Procrastination can also be described as "postponing what should be done deliberately and habitually." Too many people fool themselves into thinking that "desisting" happens only without any human intervention or involvement. This is not true, however. You must participate actively to procrastinate. If you know what has to be done and you chose not to do so, you participate actively and cause your own loss.

Imagine if you thought your body was not functioning properly and decided to see your doctor. Your appointment arrives and you have been putting it off because you thought you had worked hard all week long and you needed a bit of rest. One day turns to one week, one week to one month, and you just fail to go at all. Once you have gone to bed, you find that you have a problem that could have been stopped if you had done what was necessary. Don't let your hopes of success be destroyed by procrastination.

There is no perfect remedy but to take action. If necessary, the only solution for procrastinations is to take the necessary action. Most people go to the gym or work out, but report feeling better after they go to the gym or workout.

If you procrastinate, you feel guilty and sometimes even discouraged. People who lack the ability to perform only basic tasks have been found to be manually depressed or borderline depressed. After you have done things, you will always feel better.

Procrastination leads to stress which can lead to bad health, poor relationships, low grades and poor working performance, which can contribute to loss of employment. Nobody wants to experience these things, so why are they going on?

The first step in overcoming procrastinations is to recognize that procrastinations exist. Until you first know that you have a problem, you can't achieve "victory." It's like a medical problem. You cannot seek the appropriate care unless you "first" understand and diagnose the problem, you can then continue to treat the problem.

Discover "why" you're stuck

Knowing the "reason" behind your regression takes you closer to resolving it. Let's presume you are postponing your home cleaning. Maybe it's because you let it get out of hand that it's overwhelming to you and you just want to get away.

In general, procrastination occurs when the task that needs to be done is not pleasurable. Many people have no trouble doing things that are pleasurable for them. We are meant to move away from pain and draw near to pleasure.

Stages to combat procrastination

Stage # 1

Mind shifting: because you recognize that humans are wired to move away from painful things, this results in procrastination which is the consequence of not doing important things. Your mind creates a mental picture of the negative result if you do not do things. This mental shift can motivate you to "act" to prevent the pain of the consequences.

Stage # 2

Prioritize: You can often procrastinate because it feels as though there is too little time to do things. One way to solve this form of procrastination is by prioritizing. Specify a "to-do" list to see what the most important tasks are. Then rank the tasks according to the degree of importance (1. the most important and 10. the least important).

Stage # 3 Move

Accountability Partner: Another perfect way to counter procrastination is to nominate someone to keep you accountable. We generally strive to do what we say because we know someone else is looking at us and keeping us responsible.

Stage # 4 Prepare ahead:

This move can be linked to stage # 2. Set your "to do" goal list the night before. Completing your list in advance can first of all boost your confidence, as you've done something. You may be better able to sleep at night waiting for the next day. Since we can't predict tomorrow's events with certainty, be prepared to make any adjustments, if necessary, to your list.

CHAPTER 2

THE PROBLEM OF PROCRASTINATION

Recently I have been thinking a lot about procrastination, both its triggers and potentials. What are some of the causes? I have discovered more than a few in my exploration, but there are two that contribute to it: perfectionism and impulsivity.

With perfectionism, procrastination most times arises solely because the perfectionist cannot either start or complete a task because the result never meets the unrealistic standards of the perfectionist.

Makes sense?

The impulsive person does not have the ability to buckle down and really concentrate on anything at once. It's the principle of procrastination called "shiny thing." The impulsive tilting machine may have too many projects at once or create new ones on a fly to avoid the unpleasant work.

How well, therefore, does "perfectionism" and "impulse" explain the phenomenon of procrastination?

Let's begin with perfection.

Does perfectionism cause procrastination?

Surely it does ... To various degrees. Some people are more

affected than others. This, of course, leads directly to the problem with this theory: not all are perfectionists. But, to some degree, everybody procrastinates. This does not mean that perfectionism is the whole story.

How about the procrastination caused by impulsivity?

This is just as fair, but I don't think it explains all the hypocrisy. Imagine a deterioration that lasts months or years — impulsivity cannot easily justify this. There is real dedication to this sort of procrastination.

You've got to work hard on it, paradoxically! No, impulsivity is just one aspect of the tale of procrastination.

The Heart of Crushing

The more I look, the more it becomes apparent that procrastination is similar to cancer. There are as many kinds and perceptions of procrastinations, but they are grouped under a single umbrella.

The cause of procrastination is possibly not rooted in any psychological trait such as perfectionism or impulsiveness. It would be nice to identify one particular cause, but it's not that easy. It's not "caused" by anything, per se — it's part of who and what we are. It's an intrinsic characteristic of mankind. In fact, I think that the heart of the decline lies in our very evolution as a species; that is why the decline affects everybody.

You see, people have not been wired for long-term planning. The climate of our nomadic ancestors has provided no incentive to prepare much beyond a few weeks to a couple of months in the future. Their plans tend to be short-term or threatening, with immediate or almost immediate reward as payoffs.

Although this gives some credit to the theory of "impulsiveness" behind procrastination, it is also clear that people are able to pursue long-term strategies. As a species, it is just not our strong suit. My point is that it isn't enough time to search for its "causes". There is an endless supply of explanations for it.

It is better to determine whether you have a particular issue in one of the two specific categories of procrastinations.

Simple Procrastination versus Chronic Procrastination

I distinguish between two different "types": simple and chronic.

Simple procrastination is the kind where you are simply reluctant to do it because it's tedious or uncomfortable or bad. It can be adequately clarified by, for example, inadequate management of the momentum or excellence or inability to carry out long term planning.

A variety of approaches can resolve basic procrastination, some of which I will explain below.

What about persistent procrastinations – such as the postponed filing of taxes for years to come, or the inability to complete a fairly unassailable home improvement project for the entire summer? This form of repression takes months or years and can even destroy lives.

It is overwhelming and is a source of great stress and most attempts to resolve it are resisted. I believe that the root of chronic declination is a "disturbed" or some form of low-level fear. Whether you're consciously aware of it or not, this feeling arises, whether it makes sense even to feel that way.

In other words, the target of persistent procrastinations, such as high taxes and an unfinished project, are considered a big challenge and cause a deep instinctual drive to avoid it.

Chronic procrastination can be the product of a perceived threat to life. In other words, the mind simply correlates it with imminent death, whatever it is.

Death & Taxation

Does the mind in fact mean something unpleasant, such as finally paying overdue taxes, to death? I assume it does for the chronic procrastinator. What some find awkward, others view as a tragedy. For example, some people would prefer to be water boarded than to speaking before a live audience. Anything just as terrible as death (in the brain) appears to be fundamentally wrong in everything. Not just inaccurate, but profoundly mistaken or completely incompetent.

Have you ever felt like that?

Would you do anything to not face your peers' ridicule? It seems to me that constant isolation and absolute avoidance is a common form of dread. In some way the brain has linked chronic procrastination — overdue taxes, in the example above — to a massive penalty. In fact, there is a massive penalty that may result directly from a failure to pay taxes!

So why does the tax collector tend to make things worse by not solving the problem?

I just don't believe there is a "true" reason for chronic procrastination, except for a reasonable explanation like depression or anxiety. The patient will feel like they can't do anything; they are powerless or unable to make any progress. It is pure paralysis of motivation-a feeling of profound inner conflict and sometimes incapacity to even recognize the problem.

And what should we do with both pedestrian and omnipresent procrastinations?

Well, if my above suggestions are right, we can only assume that we can reduce procrastinations. When the declination happens as it is genetically engineered into our genes, there is no 'cure' except in a few million more years, maybe not even then.

A mitigating approach that many people turn to is technological: productivity applications, organizational structures such as GTD and other "hacks." This works for you because it works. On the other hand, it can only assist with short-term procrastinations. Chronic procrastination is a question too large for productivity hacks.

Another alternative is to use negative (punishment) motives. It is the brute-force method of resolving procrastinations, and it works for some time. An example of negative motivation is to make a promise to give money to the most despised political party if you fail to do a certain job.

How about healthy motivation?

Second, if you were already optimistic, procrastination would not be a concern. So, is there a way, so to speak, to "produce" positive motivation?

Can you be positively motivated to do something, even if you don't start like this originally?

I guess there is. For starters, once you have started a mission, it is easier to retain momentum. Yes, it really starts to feel good when continuing to work on a job or a mission, even when this is not a topic you want. Humans are set up such that it becomes easier to work on a project after it has started, as a Kenneth McGraw study reveals.

Many of the above solutions work very well for simple procrastination. Chronic procrastinations are clearly a harder nut to crack because of how omnipresent and consuming they are. For starters, against a tax-advocate you can't use much negative motivation — they already face tough fines or even prison time!

How much more can negative motivation be applied?

But with these possible penalties, they are procrastinating. To say the least, it would be unlikely if you bought a productivity app for your iPhone. Positive motivation is also not so much a consideration if the listener is consistently resistant to attempts to address the subject equally.

How to Advance Procrastination

Not all hope is lost. I believe both simple procrastinations and chronic procrastinations can be "treated" by improving attention control and meta-cognition.

If you get in touch with and concentrate on issues that cause you to be withdrawn — issues you might not even realize yet — you can at least boost your odds. At best, the challenges you once considered insurmountable can be solved. There are various ways to train your attention. The Pomodoro technology will slowly reinforce your commitment and establish good working practices.

Though I feel I might have a man-with-a-hammer syndrome, meditation is a great way to both exercise concentration and improve metacognition. You are conditioned to see the chat box in your mind that distracts you, scares you and begs for immediate gratitude. It allows you to know that no matter how compelling or seductive, you have to obey these orders.

Meditation also allows you to change your feelings and become conscious of the patterns and circumstances that can contribute to them. I have found myself less attached to certain thoughts and emotions while meditating, although they may be compelling. In spite of finding it frustrating or stressful, I find it easier to work on anything for weeks or months.

More to the point, meditation helped me to tackle frequent procrastinations on certain subjects, which was a great relief.

CHAPTER 3

PROCRASTINATION

IS IT PURE LAZINESS OR ARE WE PREDISPOSED TO PUTTING THINGS OFF?

For one, I am guilty of suffering and generally think of myself as lazy. But one night, as I lay on the couch, I thought of my busy day – I needed this excuse for not beginning my very important writing project.

I understood that I was essentially not lazy at all, that my day was full, I achieved many goals and did the work that needed attention. I just postponed the very work that was very important to me, however.

Why?

The only thing I've learned in my quest for answers is that I'm not alone. I've watched my partner and friends closely and I've discovered that most people go some similar way.

The degree to which individuals continue to procrastinate varies from the most persistent degeneration that never appears to do something for a variety of 'healthy' actual or imaginary reasons to the mild procrastinator, who can at least admit and notice when procrastination occurs and do something about it.

Why do we postpone important tasks by procrastination?

I found it most confusing. My mission was important to me, I was ready and willing, but I never felt that I was in the right mood. The phone rings and I'd better reply or what?

Why did I find something else so much more important than what I wanted?

The definition of procrastination in the dictionary is: postponement, especially out of habitual carelessness or laziness. Thus, procrastination generally refers to the act of replacing high priority acts with low-priority activities and thus postponing essential tasks until later. That's just what I was doing; after all, I wasn't lazy or was I?

A procrastinator must answer "why the mission is being procrastinated." The only reason is the incentive to take action and complete the errant task.

Essentially, procrastination is a time thief. Experts in time management can say "to write a list" and tick it as you go, but if you are like me, I can tick things off and yet skip the one thing that is really important, because it will obviously get on tomorrow's list. However, as another morning arrives, other things still seem to take precedence.

This is not the way Procrastinators are born. They have been made over time. In the family and in the school of life, we can learn the habit of procrastination. Yet I don't believe explicitly, that it's a more practiced behavior of placing pressure or concern over failure.

Why Are We Not Paying 'No Attention' To Really Critical Tasks?

Believe it or not, procrastinators tell themselves lies. They don't see themselves in their real light, they say things like, "I'm going to feel more like doing it tomorrow" or, they say, "I'm going to work the best after a good night's sleep." Moreover, they justify themselves by saying "this is not so important." In reality, procrastinators waste their resources.

There are many ways to self-sabotage your success in life, and procrastination is a choice of path people follow without even realizing it. A predictive conduct may be taken to prevent fear of failure or even fear of success.

Some people are very worried about what others think of them; others would rather believe they lack commitment rather than capacity. By not taking decisions, they take no responsibility for the outcome of events.

There can be major costs for replenishment. Health is both one and a productive life. Failure may lead to guilt, stress and insomnia which may lead to severe loss of personal productivity and a strain in personal relationships. This helps to transfer the burden of guilt to those who may then become resentful. It is therefore very important to try to change or reduce this behavior. You can change this dominant and self-sabotaging behavior.

The following traits have historically been related to procrastination:

• Perfectionism that tends to evaluate results and performance negatively.

• Intense distrust and avoidance of others' evaluation of one's abilities.

• Increased social self-awareness and fear,

• Negative mood recurring.

Exploring why you escape is the first step to a transition. Of example, there may be several reasons; fear, hate, stresses, boredom and obligation avoidance. This habit has developed for a long time, so it takes time to change. You can change your conduct; just don't expect it to change overnight.

You can experiment with different strategies as not everyone has the same strategy.

Use these helpful tips:

• Divide into smaller chunks big tasks or projects.

• Reward yourself for small achievements – you deserve it

• If you do, don't blame yourself. You will gradually develop new behaviors with new self-confidence and accomplishment feelings.

• If you find this very difficult to find, ask the 'Anti-Procrastinator Mentor,' usually a really good guy, who will warn you when you have discontinued.

• Start with your important day FIRST task and continue with all of the less important day's tasks later.

In short, most people are not lazy, but can do all kinds of things to avoid – the 'important job' of our time. It is done for a variety of reasons, most of which are not excuses, but apologies. I know it is not always deliberate to be a self-confessed procrastinator, but once accepted, you now have the power to pause and remedy.

The way to "resolve" the question of procrastination is in my view, to reap the benefit not by postponing the 'important task' but by postponing the 'less important tasks' that can be unresolved. Such success feelings are the feelings that will motivate you to improve your behavior.

CHAPTER 4

WHY PROCRASTINATION CAN BE VERY DANGEROUS TO YOUR HEALTH?

If you find yourself repeatedly procrastinating important tasks, then you are not alone. In fact, many people do not do so in different ways, but some are constantly being affected by procrastinations that stop them from fulfilling their prospects and disrupt their performance.

Procrastination is as sexy as harmful. When you think you're bored, you have to find out why you're doing it. So, once you know the explanation behind your fall, you may want to learn how to overcome it.

A simple example is a college student who does not know how to prioritize things and his program. He will invest a lot of time in RPG games or in a film marathon and he doesn't even know that next week's exam will take place.

He would push his lessons over and over, you know, tomorrow's habit and when the day before his term examination comes, he scans pages of his notes, cluttering them. He'd say to himself, it's now or never or at least I've read it, right? The result is obvious, he's going to fail. After that, he would blame himself.

Another case is that an employee who has been fired many times because she was unable to do a job, she feels very depressed and sick. Her life has been full of half-started and half-finished projects, which have led her to believe that she is extremely inept and reckless. The stress was amazing because it influenced her performance, her home life and every aspect of her life. Procrastination actually destroyed her, and she had to find a solution.

Below are several reasons why you can have poor procrastination habits and it can be very dangerous for your safety.

Personal conditions

Did you know that your personal life is not fine with procrastination?

If you repeatedly reverse household tasks or relationship duties, such as laundry, cooking, garbage taking and disposal, your marriage life and other relationships may suffer. You may then realize that declining is definitely bad if you're close to your spouse because of what you haven't taken seriously.

Don't give you inner peace

Another reason why procrastination is bad is that it removes your inner peace. Terms and meetings are always late; you run out the door, put makeup in your car, call or text on the road while driving and potentially lose your life and the people with you.

It might seem as if it is easy to postpone dental appointments, but when your cavity gets worse and you miss a day of work with your important sales presentation, you drop this customer and your promotional expectations, then you would realize how bad you are.

Hurts your reliability

Yes, your reliability or credibility is hurt by procrastination. If your friend wants something from you, your character can be so exhausted that at times she doesn't count on you to do a job.

Your best friend may have got sick and she has to get her son out of childcare school, but she might think twice before she asks you for the favor because she knows you're not punctual or will be indecisive until the school is almost over.

Provided here are measures which you can use to manage and monitor the procrastination habits:

Step 1: Understand that you are waiting

There are some symptoms and signs that allow you to recognize when you are discontinuing:

• You usually perform low-priority activities on your day.

• Reading e-mails over and over without even understanding how or whether to start interacting with them.

• Miss an element for a long time on your to-do list, although it is significant.

• Sit before your computer or desk to start a high-priority task and almost immediately make a cup of tea.

• You accept regularly non-important tasks that others want you to do and you spend your time there rather than working with the most important ones on your list.

• Normally waiting for the appropriate time or mood to execute the important task.

Step 2: Figure out why you're stuck

• Often an uncomfortable or stressful task may be the reason for your procrastination because you are trying to stop it. Finish this quickly to resolve it so you can move on and focus on the more enjoyable aspects of the task.

• Another explanation may be because you're not coordinated. The easiest way to deal with this is to make your own to-do lists and plans and prioritize them.

• Perfectionists are usually discontinued because they tend to believe that they do not have the capabilities or the resources to accomplish the task perfectly.

Stage # 3: Adopt anti-crashing methods

Procrastination is a hard-to-kill habit. Here are some important arguments to step forward:

• You must make your own incentives just like offering yourself a piece of delicious dessert chocolate cake once your mission is done. Make sure you know how good it is to finish things.

• Peer pressure really works. You may ask a friend or colleague to search. It is the concept behind self-help programs and is generally recognized as a highly successful strategy.

• The effects of not completing the job will be seen.

So, this is the fury of decline. It affects your performance, is risky, too stressful for your safety, and can sometimes be very difficult for your friends and colleagues to deal with. If you really think you're a bugger, then you need it and you must beat it immediately. So, do what you need to do today – do it now.

CHAPTER 5

THE MOST COMMON REASONS PEOPLE POSTPONE TAKING ACTION

Procrastination makes it ineffectual for you to excel in your life and career. It can be very costly. The ability to resolve it makes it easier for people to escape and then to devote themselves to being successfully. There are main reasons why you procrastinate;.

You're bored.

When life becomes routine, you just pass through the movement. When a company's initial enthusiasm weakens, most people need a new challenge. You have these easy questions to ask yourself.

Am I sick with what I do?

1. Why do I get bored?

What's going to give me more energy?

You must know that you're lonely and very aware of your feelings. Successful people are searching for greater and easier ways of keeping their juices going. The lure of a daily company is rarely something that they can fix.

2. You're frustrated by the work.

"Too many irons in the fire can cause you to degenerate." If you cause things to pile up, put it off until the next day. You are unsure how to complete your assignments. Once you are inefficient, then it becomes a twin jeopardy

There are simple steps you can take to get over it. A determined person moves quickly from one job to another because he doesn't want to leave something afterwards.

3. Your trust has slipped.

Fear and doubt lead to procrastination. If you don't know that you can do a job, inaction happens. Doubting yourself slips your confidence. If your confidence slips, then the old structures of beliefs begin to slide into your mind. Your ideas dictate your fate. When your outlook is pessimistic, the future will be pessimistic.

4. You have a low value for yourself.

Low self-esteem is a fall from the slip of confidence. If you have no self-worth, sometimes you sabotage your performance the closer you get to it. You feel that you deserve no success because of a system of negative beliefs or traumatic past.

If you have a prophecy that fulfills itself, your words will come back to you with love, desire and concentration. Success in life and industry only refers to those who really want it.

5. You do a job you just don't like.

Successful people do not do what they fail to do. Often your company allows you to perform earthly activities, such as paperwork. Often these tasks are an important part of your company.

The best thing to do is focus on the items that are perfect and outsource the rest. You 're never going to love anything you do to strike the right balance.

6. You're easily distracted, or even pitiful!

This is the leading promoter of procrastination. You don't have any problem, if you're looking for an excuse not to do something. Success takes continuous and enduring action and the equation has no legitimate place for laziness.

7. The fear of failure.

Most people don't begin a project because they fear failure. My favorite quote on this particular subject is "A thousand-mile journey starts with the first move." Never beginning you, you would never know if you had succeeded, and for the rest of your life you would regret it. Don't think about disappointment. The greatest teacher is Failure.

The fear of success is a less popular but obvious cause of procrastination. In short, I 'd be very surprised if you realized that this was your faulty reason. It's a profound anxiety that most people can't comprehend.

If you know that you are afraid of success, you have to look at why you are afraid of success. You are probably just afraid of change, and if the project succeeds, it will change your life.

8. Not really motivated by the topic or possible results.

The most common reason why people are not motivated to start is by far not enough. It can be used for so many things. For example, a student in school might not really feel motivated to get a good degree and go to a good college. Such pay offs are highly remote and immaterial.

It is difficult to be motivated by a reward too far away. Another example is that you don't care about the job you have. You definitely won't feel inspired if you think that the job is pointless or uninteresting.

9. There is no time limit.

Deadlines are one of the key reasons why people know that they have a problem with procrastination. A time limit requires you to rest and get your job done. But if you don't have a deadline, you can carry on until you are gone. Long deadlines are the worst cause of procrastination and the absence of deadlines is a major reason for people to procrastinate.

10. We have better / more important things to do

For example, let's work out and get in shape. I still try to inspire people who have little time to practice and I always get the same excuse. "I'll start a program in the near future, but I've got too many important tasks on my platform."

If it doesn't matter to you in your life, why do you even pretend to? Nobody says you have to do it perfectly or spend an unreasonable amount of time in the practice, just start!

Everything you need to do is important; you can always spend time on another important activity, even if it is only 10 or 15 minutes.

11. We're not "owed" to start

Some people fall into the "full planning" mode. We put it off because they don't feel prepared enough.

The truth is, the best way to train yourself for any activity is to practice it. The things that we believe are "necessary" for a certain task or activities are so often superfluous that we can benefit by starting NOW with a small change.

Again, take the example (hey, I AM Mr. Fat Loss ... what did you expect?)

There are people who say they cannot be put in shape because their gym membership has expired, or they can't find the correct personal trainer, or they have to buy a new pair of running shoes to start playing again ... BS! Take your chest and pushup ... no MATTER WHERE YOU ARE! It's an excuse ... nothing more.

12. We are too busy

We're so busy; The difference is in the types of work we do that keeps us occupied. When we handle time effectively, almost all of us could find the time needed to start the tasks that we put off. If we wait for a while before beginning another task or project, this time may never come.

You always have to do things; the key is how you organize your time. This explanation is close to operation number one. Using the "too busy" excuse generally means you filled your day with "things." You didn't have time to begin this new training program because you were at the movies or you were sitting in the couch with a friend at lunch. That's a pretext, not a reason.

Stop twisting and resume twisting. Through listing your regular activities, you will continue to add your FIRST activities and make them part of your everyday routine. When you know that an activity is successful, do not offer a "reason" to do so, build an OPPORTUNITY that you can start doing!

Even if a goal is not accomplished, the effort is in itself a reward. Good learning comes through experience, which can only be done through practice. Moreover, most citizens consider and support a brave initiative regardless of the result. The attempt is an act of courage. The avoidance is central to cowardice. Do not fall into the pit of using fear as an excuse for degeneration.

13. Feeling overwhelmed and exhausted.

We sometimes look at a goal and believe like so much need to be achieved to accomplish it. The feeling that we are overwhelmed paralyzes us and prevents us from taking even the first step towards our objective.

Break it into different pieces for each goal you have in life. Determine what actions are needed for each component to succeed. If you look at the big picture and feel overwhelmed, then, look at the little steps along the road. Take them one by one, without the next worrying. Move ahead with every individual win and you will have found success before you know it.

14. Human nature.

Naturally, we prefer to avoid what causes us trouble or discomfort, and we step towards what is simple or fun. In order to prevent distress due to the uncomfortable or challenging nature of a task, attempt first to do the most stressful work.

Immerse yourself in a can-do mentality and know that the sooner you begin and the more difficult you work, the sooner it is over. To deal with the most difficult tasks paves the way first for smoother sailing along the coast.

15. The viewpoint.

When we find a mission to be challenging, this is exactly what it is for us. Rather than fearing a given job, see it as an opportunity to succeed. If you are asked to complete a research mission, see it as the chance to learn new knowledge and to extend your intellectual limits. You can turn a chore into fun by plunging into a project with passion, wherever it is located. Take a look to see if it helps to fan the flames of excitement.

Throughout history, there has been much talk about the destructive nature of procrastination. Some of the easiest ways to do this is to forget what fate we will have tomorrow, because we arc better positioned to feel what we can now.

Another irony is that too many of us lament about not having ample time to sit idly, ignoring the job that is waiting for us. If we just dug our hands and started, the day would probably be longer, and we'd accomplish much more.

If you find it difficult to achieve your objectives, take a look at the steps you have to take to succeed and ask yourself whether you have fallen into the dark tree of repulsion. Examine your own reasons for procrastinating, then promise yourself you won't let it kill your hopes and dreams.

16. Feeling anxious and stressed

When you feel depressed, nervous or exhausted, it may be very difficult to get productive. Some people also procrastinate as a way to cope with and maintain control over stress. The best way to overcome stress is to spend enough time relaxing and having fun.

As the old saying goes, "Playing and no playing will make you a dumb and stressful guy." You also need to invest ample time for relaxation and recreational activities. Then use whatever time remains to do your job. You don't have to put off your work in that way, because you think you have to have fun and relax.

Be very careful, however, when using this strategy. You could spend your entire time enjoying yourself and forget your job absolutely. What you have to do is share the time for yourself and your family properly.

17. Working more than you can take on issues.

Sometimes there are just too many things that cannot be done on your to-do list. Then you will feel easily overwhelmed, which can also lead to procrastination. It's like your brain refuses to work on a very unreasonable schedule. If this is the case, your to-do list may need to be rewritten. Specify your goals and remove something that is not relevant.

18. Laziness.

In certain instances, when a person feels physically or emotionally exhausted, a person appears to feel lazy and sometimes people are just purely lazy and try to do their homework as soon as possible. Even the easiest tasks can seem difficult for lazy people so they continue to procrastinate.

It is because their energy is too small relative to the amount of energy needed for the mission. The solution is quite straightforward. You will snap out of your faintheartedness. A healthy lifestyle, diet and exercise will also help increase your energy.

CHAPTER 6

WHY HAVING A TO DO LIST DOES NOT WORK AND WHAT TO DO ABOUT IT?

What's a "to do list?"

I find it to be fairly clear that a "to do list" should identify all the things that you will perform for a certain period of time.

If people start making lists and planning their tasks, they are more likely to procrastinate, why?

That's because you know you have a lot of work ahead of you to finish a project or something that requires a series of steps to finish.

What do people usually do when they see a lot of things coming along?

If it is really a number, our mind cannot manage everything, and we 'ignore' something else: other unproductive tasks that waste even more energy. It is important to note that a "to do list" is simply a method for organizing your tasks and activities but does not mean that they are completed or finished.

Action is required to remove from the list tasks and activities.

The reason why "to do lists" do not work is because it takes time to make them and also, as I said, usually we do not work when we see big work piles before us (this is what a list emphasizes). The longer the list of things to do, the more work it entails, and therefore

38

the idea that we have a lot of work causes us to pause.

So, what should I do?

Set up a list of "what to do!"

You will write in this list the things you will NOT consider because these activities have not helped you in any way because of previous experience. You will sit down and reflect for a few minutes to recognize things you shouldn't do. This can be linked to any time or any day.

Example: you can explain things that you don't have to do only in the morning. The example may be that at night you don't have those activities.

It is particularly useful if you know where you're doing your best during the day. If you work best during the morning you may want to describe the "not to do list" for this specific time with all unproductive activities. If you set it as a personal rule, and keep all commitments for yourself, your job will be even more successful because the "no list" will allow you to postpone all unproductive activities.

Let me explain a specific example to stress what I mean.

Let's say, in the morning I work at my best. That is when I'm calm and there are not so many breaks. At night, before I go to bed, I explain all the unproductive things that I don't have to do in the morning or when I wake up, which steal my energy and my focus.

My "not to be mentioned" tasks typically includes e-mail

searches, social media reviews, no morning coffee drinks, no morning smoking, no morning surfing on different websites, which could take me away from my job and no morning shopping with friends.

I can now focus on what is important when I write down those "no activities" and do this until they are complete. You must identify activities that give you the highest return on your investment and all activities that keep you unproductive.

You will have more control over your productive working habits and eventually do things much faster when you commit to yourself and write them on a paper in all the things you should not do in a particular period.

How to Cut Back To-Do Lists

Often, I wonder why procrastination is such a major issue. After all, we live in a productivity-obsessed society. Everyone needs to do this more and more efficiently, in less time.

Companies are cutting roles and asking employees to do two (or more) jobs. Parents prepare each moment of their child's life and both have expectations and aspirations to achieve.

With such an attempt to be always successful, there should not even be a prolongation of language as a term. And yes, even if we have all read productivity books, subscribed to websites and tried tools for managing time, we never seem to be done enough.

Perhaps it is because we expect so much of ourselves. I end with a 16-hour day as I map my days with everything on my to-do lists. I'm trying to control my expectations, but I'll inevitably get rid of everything I * need * and eventually have three days in a row watching the whole season of the TV show feeling like a total loser.

Fortunately, I figured it out and now I know the stresses that tell me to look at my expectations prior to the meltdown. I have learned why I procrastinate and use these reasons to decide what I'm going to cut down from my list and clear my habits.

There are three reasons why we procrastinate (for me):

Lack of interest: we just don't want to do what we are asked to do

Inertia: an inaction pattern prevents us from starting.

Fear: failure, success, conflict with the right people or satisfy the wrong

Let us look at each of these explanations to see if we can use them to find out exactly where our goals can be calculated.

Lack of Interest

It's the best if you look at a task and you think "m'eh" or "blue!" why are you doing it??

What if you just crossed it off your list?

Would the world crumble? Very unlikely.

So, if you want to do it, you are the right person to do it? Would you find someone else to do that?

The first time we do something new, it costs us a lot more energy and effort than the tenth time we do it.

Fear

I think there are two kinds of fear. One is our intuition that this is the wrong path and get away before we go into a car. The other is our deepest wishes whisper in our hearts and we are in the top of a roller coaster because of the thrill of terror.

How are we told the difference?

Okay, the first is a garbage, while the second is a rubbing-heart wheel! If it's the first, then drop anything you do as soon as you can. If it is the second, pursue it with all your might.

Look at your schedule now. Write down what you want to do. Label all the things with D (for disinterest), I (for inertia) or F (for fear). Cut off or assign the tasks of yourself, prioritize and schedule the tasks of depression and find ways to make your fears thrill. When you have done this, you will have a to-do list, and that will be a thing of the past.

The Roots of Procrastination

The difference between the winner and the loser lies in the way they live, because their future lies in your everyday routines. Habits-predict and shape your future.

Procrastination is the usual practice of postponing an action or to avoid an essential activity until later. It is the tendency to wait before taking action for the perfect condition. But unfortunately, if such a perfect condition does not come, you will do nothing.

When not stopped, this activity would harm and impede your career growth, harm your relationship and wellbeing, keep you from pursuing what you really want and ultimately make you feel depressed and unfulfilled. Slack habits are as vandalistic as they are!

In accordance with the "Cause and Effect" rule, replacement can be seen and seen as the result of certain causes, which I called the roots of replacement. Invariably, these roots, the reasons, provide the necessary nourishment for procrastination unconsciously.

Unbelievably, the majority of us still are not able to recognize these factors and it is also impossible for us to resolve this given our struggle to live without interruption. Nevertheless, before being a chronic replacement, I will unveil some of the roots of replacement and how they are eradicated. Read on! Read on!

1. Lack of preparation and ignorance

"Ignorance is a disease," they claim, and chance meets the ready mind. Procrastination is one of the signs of this disorder. Ignorance is the lack of appropriate knowledge to help you unlock an idea.

Owing to your lack of intelligence, your lack of knowledge, your indifference or your unpreparedness, you cannot now implement and handle the great ideas that come to mind.

You can't write a proposal for a business, start your own business, etc. The excuse is I'm not ready. Try to look back at all the opportunities you have put off if there is a lack of preparation or information. If there are any, ask yourself that question:

When will I be prepared and better informed?

You need to search for more knowledge to eliminate ignorance and lack of planning. I decided once to implement an idea I had. It's all about how other individuals and organizations overcome a problem. But I didn't know how to do it. The reality is that if you don't have the details, you will not be interested, so that you cannot be involved and no action will be taken.

Read newspapers, books, internal papers, speak to people who you feel are willing to get facts and do research. Get acquainted with what you need. Familiarity leads also to curiosity.

2. Fear.

Fear trembles before what you face and when you trembled, you stopped seeing what you face. Everyone has everyday ideas and opportunities, which make us stand out and let our name be the profile of successful people in our generation if well used and done. It's the fear of failure for some of us, probably because we have previously failed.

Failure does not mean that you're weaker, you're wasting your time or never going to do something; it just offers an opportunity for you to demonstrate your dominance, learn something new and make it better when you start up again.

How often did you avoid or postpone doing something because of fear?

Fear of making mistakes?

I discovered that nothing can cripple a man more than fear, because even the physically crippled can be manipulated medically to drive a car by using artificial legs, but a full fearful man with 2 legs may not be a passenger and therefore will not change his position.

In order to overcome fear, you need:

I) Identify the cause of your fears;

II) Learn from the knowledge of your past;

III) Develop courage and deal with your fears;

IV) Try to start doing what you are afraid of, and what you fear will disappear; the fears will no longer be later or sooner.

3. Distraction

Distractions are unexpected interruptions that require your time to be additional and annoying. You have to sideline yourself and lose concentration and change the attention from what you actually do. A lot of distractions will help you go a long way.

Many of those who procrastinate are also easily distracted in most situations. Most of this distracts us at times from our daily routines like watching TV, listening to a conversation at the next office, asking who walks down the stairs and so forth. Create a list of the things that confuse you easily and reflect if you procrastinated by doing these things.

To avoid distraction, you have to:

I) Prepare what you plan to do that day in writing and reflect on why you plan to do these things before the start of the day. Planning contributes to practice directly

II) Keep the TO DO LIST before you or remember it. If you keep it in front of you, you can choose what to do next.

III) Remove or avoid all potential distracting stimuli around you.

IV) Ask yourself what my time is best for now. This keeps you focused and increases your concentration certainly on what you can do in your TO DO LIST.

The most common reasons for procrastination are lack of preparation and information, fear and distractions. Such factors always create one reason or the other to never act or decide.

However, it is undoubtedly believed that your commitment and zeal to find solutions to each of these causes will help you in your efforts to overcome procrastination.

CHAPTER 7

HOW TO CREATE AN ACTION-PROMPTING REWARD SYSTEM TAILORED TO YOUR PERSONAL PROCLIVITIES

In this chapter I want to set the stage for further discussion of the importance of rewards. First, it's important to let yourself think more positively.

We seem eager enough to shout at ourselves and judge ourselves harshly if we do not fulfill a task or goal which we have set for ourselves. This is often a custom we have learned from others who have been preaching it.

For balance purposes only, you may want to add some reward to the mix and see how much more you're doing and how much better you feel. For many of us, it seems all too tempting to envision the worst. The worst-case scenarios just occur as quickly as if we had spent a lot of time and effort psychologically confirming them.

Now, what if you took some of your precious time and energy and get started

Concentrate on something more effective.

The subconscious minds are aware that what really is possible, what we need, what we want and really different from reality. The more true and vivid you can do things in your mind, the easier it will be as long as you think that, at least on a certain level, it is possible.

This influential part of our minds will tell you what a safe and useful visualization towards achievable targets is and help you understand how to get there more quickly and efficiently. While mere mental masturbation may not be the worst thing, it is rather a pleasant waste of time.

However, the worst-case scenario is an even worse waste of your precious time and energy because these potentially dangerous chemicals will still be released into our corpora. The only way to escape worry is to schedule and be prepared! The needless extra stress of negative thinking is not only necessary but can also cause potential harm.

Strong and pessimistic self-talking will make the body immune and defense systems very uncomfortable. The additional burden will affect our health and will certainly affect our best functionality.

Therefore, continue to devote at least some time and energy to more practical and, probably, more optimistic views and tests. It's like feeding a certain kind of food to your stomach. It may take a while to get there.

Positive thoughts allow the door to be opened and are often the most important step toward your goals. Having a positive outlook and then finding out what steps you need to take to achieve these objectives.

You will face obstacles and difficulties along the way, and you will benefit from the actions you take. This critical input is important for learning, development and performance.

A failure gives up too quickly and easily and we cannot all be motivated entirely by ourselves. This is where coaching is at stake. People really like someone to give them ideas.

Anyone will ask you to do your utmost, and then you can ask yourself (where to make a half-hearted effort is more like saying you have done and not putting your best foot forward really)

The "to do list" can help to clear up your everyday tasks and make room for things you want to do to make your goals closer. Many people are distracted or monitored on the side by day's activities, and this method will allow you "to do things"

Return now to what I mean by right and wrong actions. False claims or actions destroy your chances of achieving your goals, or at best waste your precious time. The right actions or things help you to achieve your goals and the best ways to do that are to be rewarded to remain motivated.

The best way to remain motivated and accountable is to reward yourself for taking action that seems to bring you closer to your goals.

There is no real drawback or failure to act and whatever you do to get suggestions on where you have to go. It is clear that to do something that is not closer to your goals and you need to change your direction or re-evaluate your plans step by step. Some people find the willingness to do this alone, while others prefer some help and guidance and coaching.

Focus on a positive attitude every day and make a quick "list" and use it to get the boring work off the ground and clear a path to greater happiness. If you approach your destination, you will feel better that you are closer to your goals.

By taking advantage of the infinite energy of our subconscious mind, we use all our energy to achieve continued success while maintaining the necessary versatility to tackle the obstacles which life throws our way.

Wake up with a sort of zeal-like calm every morning so that the feedback can help you get closer to your objectives and continue to act decisively.

The "to do list" can help you to remove those not so exciting yet essential tasks that we all have to perform every day. This can give you more time and energy to work on your goals for greater success.

CHAPTER 8

WHY CRITICIZING YOURSELF ALWAYS LEADS TO MORE PROCRASTINATION AND WHAT TO DO INSTEAD

I used to be my worst baseball enemy. On the plate I would doubt, play timid defense and lack trust on the base paths. It was like a little man who told me how poor I was, how useless I was, how inadequate I was, how I could not succeed, how the team saw me as a liability, etc., It became so clear that I had to find a way to stop the inner critic.

Hearing your inner critic begins when you have no trust or fear to decide. In childhood sometimes it occurs, while others or we find it difficult to think positively in a steak of bad fortune. Once you interrupt this internal criticism, you will stop feeling sorry for yourself and change your feelings into positive ones.

Positive thinking is the beginning of the internal criticism. Tell yourself that you're not good, and that nobody cares, helps anyone, even yourself. You have to believe, start thinking happy thoughts and positive things will happen.

Often, we underestimate a mission, strategy or plan and it seems like an impossible task. You may first think, "I can't do this!" But if you divide the task into more small ones and put in a realistic plan, as you continue your strategy you will gain confidence.

Only a little improvement can have a huge impact on your psyche. Confidence comes with more practice; positive thinking cos with trust. Practice is how the inner criticism ends.

Another way to stop the inner critic is not to take yourself so seriously. Laugh a bit, nobody's perfect. Looking at the lighter side will help to release the stress and lift the minds.

Don't keep anything cut inside. Speak to someone, perhaps a parent, colleague, or coach. It will make you feel better and somebody will cheer you up. It is therapeutic and recommended to have an outlet to release your feelings and frustration and an excellent way to stop the inner critic.

It is a cultural phenomenon that criticism or emphasis on guilt motivates behavior. Maybe you think you won't want to improve if you know that your acts are not good enough or ideal? The critic gives us a sense of power as well.

People in our lives will make "helpful" but important observations to improve and regulate our actions and feelings. We may also use judgment or self-control as a way to cope with the anxiety, the guilt and the unknown. These remarks (both from others as well as from ourselves) internalize and become our "inner critics" over time.

Sadly, this form of contact induces fear and bullying, which ultimately does the opposite of motivation. This leads us to stop, decrease anxiety and stay healthy. Avoidance (reduce anxiety) is not equal to motivation for improvement.

Avoidance usually involves things like procrastination, addictive behavior (for instance, overfishing, grassing when not hungry, drinking, and smoking), constantly checking your mobile, watching excessive television, or even avoiding the source of criticism and/or shame (such as yourself, the action, your location, or even the person)

In fact, if words like "what's wrong with you" or "you're not good enough" are insulting, we can get paralyzed. Shame takes us apart from others and encourages us to feel lonely.

As humans, we are hardwired for communication at a cellular level. If we are scared, these emotions physically make us want to flee, withdraw and further cause preventative behaviors to reassure or relax us.

Why do you understand and let your criticism go?

Knowledge is the first move. Many of us don't even realize the inner critic's presence. Catch yourself the next time you feel nervous, depressed or dumb. Identify the inner vital voice. Identify the condition that the inner critic may have caused.

What are your genuine feelings about this?

Remember, you feel in control by the inner critic. Ask yourself, then, what do I fear?

What if that happened, what would it mean?

So, what is that going to mean?

Enable yourself to delve deeper into the situation and to find your most weak sentiments. This is what the inner critique protects you against feeling.

Do you need all this protection? Probably not. You can handle it!

Exercise: The inner critique works

1. What are those self-criticisms that you're aware of hearing you say? Explain it to the second person. E.g.: you're such a coward, you 're disgusting, you 're useless.

2. How do you feel listening to this? Touch the feeling.

3. What are some real feelings about this situation that are not related to the shameful triggers that you may have?

4. What are the reactions?

5. What are you telling that voice that says you are useless?

6. What are you really going to do about yourself? Or what are you really supposed to hear?

Tell this to your inner critic in the following steps of compassion:

1. Share concern with the interior critic's anxiety and emotions out of control: what you felt at step 3; "I understand, for example, that you are afraid of being hurt and rejected. I know that you're trying to protect me against these feelings.

2. Voice your answer (step 4). Your vital voice doesn't help, however. Don't talk to me like that, please. It prevents me from getting what I need and feeling connected to others. I'll be all right. I can cope with everything that happens.

3. What I really need (step 6) is to communicate and reach out to others. I don't have to be scared or deprive myself of fear.

Core beliefs in connection with internal criticism and negative self-discussion:

Here are some core beliefs with which the inner critic's self-talk may be associated. They are essentially in 1 out of 2 categories: the poor self or the weak self.

The wrong person is grounded in shame and the belief that you are not good enough. You may see yourself as:

-unrelenting

-Failed

- Unwanted.

-- lower and be ashamed of perceived insufficiency

- Evil and worthy of punishment, still feel guilty

-incompetent if they're not the best or not as good as others

The weak feeling of self is based on anxiety and fear and the conviction that you cannot cope and survive on your own. People may have the following convictions:

-dependent; believing that others need to survive

-unable to help yourself

-submissive; I have to put the needs of others before me

-It will lead to something bad expressing my needs or anger

-- The soul is fragile

-There will be something bad or I will lose control

The weak senses of the self are all associated with beliefs about connection, deprivation, abandonment, lack of trust and isolation.

Words used: I'm never going to get the love I like, I 'm going to be all alone, nobody ever embraces me.

Such convictions are neither helpful nor useful. In general, they are harmful. Practice listening to hints about these convictions by taking care of your inner critic's self-talk over the next few weeks. Challenge those convictions! They are not true. You are worthy, able and worthy of love.

Make Friends With Your Inner Critic

What's your critical voice saying to you?

Does it say you 're not good enough?

When you make a mistake, does it scold you?

Perhaps it means you're going to mess things up and you're never going to win, because you never have.

Your inner critic's strength could be so strong that it stops you from really living your life.

Perhaps you're not going for the job you want, because the voice says you're never going to get it. You might avoid intimate relationships or social situations, because your critic warns you against refusal. Perhaps it is that chronic whisper that causes you to

56

hide your creative projects or worse, it stops you all together from creating them.

The more you hear your vital voice, the more you trust it. You won't doubt it if you believe it and you'll constantly behave to prove your inner critic is right, because you believe it.

What if you could make friends with it instead of bowing to the power of your critical voice?

Here's what I know about the inner critic from personal and professional experience:

It recirculates ancient convictions about you.

It repeats what other people have told you.

It's not your real voice.

It tries to protect you.

You use it to stay healthy.

You are stronger than your vital voice.

Your critical voice is aimed at the exact places you most need forgiveness and compassion.

You can begin to see how your critical voice tries to protect you when you understand. For instance, it's easy to hold back when you think you're not good enough.

Holding back may seem like a good way to feel safe. Just what your vital voice wants.

Unfortunately, standing back typically sounds much worse than bravely progressing. The next time you want to stop your inner critic, take a moment to remember it. Let's stop saying, "Hello, I'm listening to you. Thank you for keeping me safe."

Next, tell it some of the encouraging words you want instead to hear. It takes time, but it will be easier and easier to believe in yourself with practice.

Transfer your courage from discouragement to encouragement.

Remember that your inner critic is focusing on your hidden and unsafe spots. These are the places in which the encouragement, the compassion and the understanding are needed. More criticism will not help – only more retention will be triggered.

EFT Tapping is a perfect tool for pivoting your critical voice.

Use EFT (Emotional Freedom Techniques) to help release the negative feelings caused by your critic. Next, tap into constructive, inspiring words using EFT.

Bottom line – you want your vital voice to keep you safe. It's sneaky and sly, and it's going to do everything to get your attention. You have to tame it. Find ways to make your risk feel safer. Techniques like EFT, meditation and guided imaging will be of assistance. Do whatever you can to make yourself look as good as you really are!

How to Silence Your Inner Critic

Everyone's inner voices have been around, in the universe, in every time period. Are you like many others who wonder how to silence your inner critic?

Whoever you are, or what you have or may not have, or even where you are, it is a natural part of the process and patterns of life to develop patterns of thought and action.

Most of this internal conviction develops from some external entity, whether elementary or in the form of another person or people. Your inner critique actually helps you in life, but as time progresses, this process develops into negativity in thinking patterns for most individuals.

Identifying your inner critic

The inner critic typically works behind the mind at the unconscious level. However, even we learn about our inner critic. Most frequently, we do not even know the possible effect it has on our everyday lives.

Whenever our inner critic focuses on a negative aspect rather than a positive one, we experience greater stress, anxiety and depression.

You can easily recognize your own inner critic as the voice that tries to lead you somehow within your mind. If you have been programmed by the negative influences of others and external elements in your sphere of existence, it is often up to you to replay much of the unnecessary and detrimental inner dialog that degrades you.

But you should be aware that you can learn how to silence your inner critic and create more positive lifestyles and patterns which will help you become who you really are while you follow the true purpose of your life.

Accept your inner critic

One of the most important steps in learning how to silence your inner critic is to recognize that it does not only exist in you, but also in others. The inner critic exists in your mind as an internal controlling voice. Everybody's got one.

Although it is a small voice, it can be focused very loudly and negatively, even though it's not the whole of your very life since it really doesn't have a place in your heart.

What does all this mean when it comes to how the inner critic can be removed? It means that we all go through it, because we all have that small internal voice to guide us. Sometimes your inner critic is enveloped by external influences and can be overwhelmingly confusing, rather than resourceful, when we draw on the negativity we can afford.

There are also many ways to help you learn how to relax and balance your mind like using items that give you the resources to conquer negativity by replacing it with constructive habits of thinking, so that better things will happen in your life.

When you are ready to find the best way to calm your inner critic and focus on the positive outlook of yourself and your life, you will have the useful resources.

Be Friends With Your Inner Critic and You Will Discover a Greater You

We all have this inner voice which often prevents us from changing. It's a fear of failure at times and a fear of success at times. It may keep us from starting a new home, meeting new challenges or learning new skills. Our inner critic often drains our energy and creates self-doubt and low self-esteem. The inner critic is like an overprotective mother who wants the best for us but keeps us in the process.

See the examples below and see if you can connect with them:

1. You may interview a potential team member and want to boost your business when you hear a voice saying, "You have already achieved success in your current career, why do you bother even?"

2. You may have just begun to call and invite friends and relatives to a presentation when the inner voice says, "Your friends are already busy with their lives.

3. You may have built a successful business, and you may be ready to quit when you hear, "That's too risky to do; in this economy, you will never do it!"

You doubt yourself because of this inner voice that damages your good ideas. It's a voice with us all day long. It tells us who we are and how we do, describes and interprets our every experience. It is very difficult to get us to recognize its interpretations as our reality.

Become a leader and look at your critic in a positive way

To be a leader, you must be aware of what events trigger your arrival as the inner critic shows up in you. Recognize how it makes you feel and how it affects your decision to move on or reverse what you really want.

Once you have observed your own inner voice, begin to recognize when your team members have the inner voice. Watch how they present their first business opportunity; there's probably your inner critic!

As a good leader, it is crucial that you recognize the presence of the inner critic and help your team member understand how it is handled. By sharing your understanding with your team members, you can help them monitor and transcend the fears and doubts created by this inner voice.

Your success and your team's success depend on your ability to transform the inner critic from adversary to friend. These six steps help you to learn how.

1. List three messages that your inner voice frequently gives and explains how these signals make you feel.

2. Give personal names, drawings or descriptions to the inner voice.

3. Choose your answers attentively. Choose to distinguish between the inner critic and the fact.

4. Affirm true strengths, achievements and qualities to reprogram negative messages of the inner voice into positive messages.

5. Have a meaningful dialog with your inner voice in order to understand and build a healthy relationship with it.

6. Be the observer; judge not. Be proactive instead of reactive.

Practice these steps and you will start developing a lighter relationship with your inner critic. Take responsibility for the way it works best for you. Gradually, you will hear the inner voice become calm and know that you are free and able to take care of yourself!

CHAPTER 9
TRICK TO BUILD "NOW HABITS" TO STOP PROCRASTINATION

Habits are what we voluntarily want or do not want. They can grow in us, they can bring us fortune, success, wealth, happiness or they can destroy our hopes, aspirations, our whole lives, the lives of family, society and nation completely. Habits can destroy the world! Our behavior determines our habits.

Procrastination is blamed on itself. It's a tradition. Let's become factual; if this statement cannot be accepted, close this page immediately!

You don't want to change your thinking, your thoughts-your being-why waste your time or bother yourself, because it is just foolish to believe you can continue to do the same as you always have and get varied results. You can be overpriced – that's the simple truth. If not, you'd not be bothered to try to find a solution.

If you decide to stop today, then you have decided to turn around your life. Changing your life, celebrating, being counted amongst historians, being the best in your field, your business, your niche, your relationship, and so forth. If you haven't, then you may only desire death for nothing. What's the point if you can't make a difference?

Interestingly, people make things happen; the revolution behind more and better apps, innovative games, concepts, spaceships, movies, medical breakthroughs... It is even better not to say that it is you, the force behind the motion, who made the impact!

The strength behind the motion will make you to stop the procrastination. Given the established consequences of knowingly postponing an expected course of action. The bad habit can be avoided by imbibing A New Habit –Now.

Highly effective people have become used to making decisions quickly and gradually, if and when they are changed. Conversely, mediocre ones decide, if at all, very slowly and as their emotions change-fast and often.

The decision to do things as soon as they are made should be taken promptly.

How often have you preferred to be the best in your field such as making new friends, washing the dishes promptly, quitting smoking, making a call for business, strengthening relations, losing some weight and starting a training plan.

How many times have you had programs, steps and plans of action designed to implement your dream?

How often did you tell yourself that you would start immediately, right now?

How often did you fail?!

Think you are no better than the other man, Gal, who never

bothered to spend his time on unsuccessful ventures-decisions that you will never take?

Who says you can never do it?

Who says that you can't bounce back?

Unless you firmly believe you could not reach the top, no force on this planet can stop you. Without your consent, nobody can make you feel less-Eleanor Roosevelt.

Nobody can make you feel defeated in the same vein except for your claim and confirmation. By instilling the following tips, we can try to stop Procrastination. Choose the one that suits you and proceed.

Next, do the boring research and forget about it.

If a task appears powerful or not inviting, the truth is that you have to do it and avoid problems in the future – break it down and tackle it bit by bit.

- Choose a time-limit on all your tasks. Make them realistic so you won't be frustrated if you can't achieve very ambitious objectives. There is a sort of pressure when a deadline is applied to a mission.

- Disregarding protocols-you just need to sometimes start something-you can start anyway, so you have the momentum to continue, and so that you can keep up with orders when you feel motivated.

- Change your understanding, change your behavior!

Since you can easily lie to and mislead your subconscious, you are your own worst enemy. What you think is what your subconscious does. You can tell your subconscious a wrong interpretation of a job and it will say-yes boss, this is exactly what it is.

So why not say good things, change your attitude and your thinking about that task — tell your subconscious and watch it say — yes, boss, that's it, and now we can!

Now consider the effect of putting an assignment off the ground, not being responsible, not in full control, not calling, not checking your dentist or physician, not trying to lose weight, stop smoking, being the leader in the market, being the best you can.

If you are a perfectionist like I was before, you must first understand that human nature is imperfect. In fact, two years ago, I postponed the start of a web business because I wanted to get it right the first time. Then I saw my ideas littering around the internet without a dent of perfection.

People, they roll in millions every year! I'm sitting here, watching and waiting for the first time, who's is losing? I'm the fool who regrets everywhere. Now I said to myself, that the information you have is enough to get you started, just go ahead-as you progress you will find out more. That's how I began. It was all out of necessity.

Start this minute, please. For you, I'm on my knees. I can't wait until you unleash a million dollars project for mankind, reconcile with the old guy, save yourself for 10 more years if you quit smoking now, look more attractive if you battle obesity right now, test your teeth with your dentist or whatever.

"I can do that tomorrow." How often do you say that both about the big and the small, important and trivial things of life?

How often do you slow down, deliberately postpone, unnecessarily procrastinate, drag your feet and usually do not act?

How many times do you postpone actions that you have to carry out? How often do you shove your dreams back out of fear of failure, faint-heartedness, or perfection? There is no doubt that the reply to each question is "Yes, sometimes" – thanks in part to human nature. Each of us is the victim of Someday, Someday, Someday Syndrome: 'I will, Someday.'

There's a better choice. Why not substitute the Someday, Someday Syndrome with a stronger, optimistic, constructive everyday habit: "Hey, I am." If you want to, you can do that, but you must admit that you have a twist, look at why, build a strategy that can improve your behavior, and create a new set of habits. You probably think "easier to say than to do," and you are right. It's easy to substitute.

When you do it, you feel like you risk nothing. When you shoot a job, activity, or dream, it's 'out of sight, out of mind.' You're not supposed to think about it. You can continue with your life and focus on things you really want to do, tasks that are more enjoyable, more pleasant and less dangerous.

However, in truth, the job you do not realize is always on your "Things to Do List," and every time you revisit your list – or worse, each time your boy or spouse tells you that this job needs to be completed – it generates a punch of concern.

You procrastinate the mission until the last possible moment to generate needless tension in the race. Unfortunately, in the case of dreams, daily life marches along, your dream goes unfulfilled, and at the end of your Earth time you end up with painful regrets for what could have been.

Rather than thinking, "Maybe I'm going to do it tomorrow," do something to improve your quality of life today. If you wait until tomorrow, maybe you will never arrive at tomorrow. It may never happen if you wait for a better time to act.

Do the best you can with your time, your talents and today's circumstances. Take a decision to stop procrastination and place your goals at the top of your priority list, as you know it will improve your life. If you need assistance, find these basic steps of common sense that will lead to a strategy that helps you to focus on today rather than waiting for tomorrow and to execute plans that never see the daylight:

- Find a quiet place to think about it, maybe your favorite coffee house or perhaps a park. Take out your notebook and put on your mind hat. Examine your daily life and habits. Make a list of all the things you are postponing, large and small.

For example: I'm going to start saving money for an emergency fund tomorrow. I'm going to plan a dream trip to Italy tomorrow. I will return to school tomorrow and finish my college degree. I'm going to write my novel tomorrow. I'm going to start a workout tomorrow. I'm going to make peace with my family tomorrow. You're getting the idea. Develop a complete list.

- Check every item on your list and ask "why" you are stopping. What is the way to start and complete each task on your list? Some tasks are obligatory, but you procrastinate: you may postpone a project, because you are fully qualified to do it, but it is not a task you enjoy, so you drag your feet. There are certain tasks that invoke fear and so you hold back.

- You are concerned that you do not have the skill or the ability to write the novel that you always dreamt about. Some tasks take lots of time and a lot of sweat equity: You may want to tackle this long list of projects for home improvement, but you do not seem to find enough time or energy.

- Some tasks involve resources that you think you don't have: maybe you'd like to start saving for retirement, but you live with a check for pay and are waiting until your finances improve. There are so many scenarios, each individual. What is important is to get a detailed picture of your life.

- Admit that you are slowing down and plan today to improve.

Make the pledge to stop twitching and replace bad habits with healthy, constructive habits: today with excitement and pride, I deal with my dreams and responsibilities.

- Recognize that you cannot tackle each item on your list immediately.

What are you able to handle right now-and finish today?

Start this task. It's a simple 'win.' Then, quickly, one by one, knock off anything that can be accomplished quickly and easily; it will shorten your list and encourage you to concentrate on a more challenging mission.

It will also send you along the path to build a new, healthier habit: proactive vs. proactive. This effort will contribute to your trust, self-esteem and momentum as you give priority to all long-term and labor-intensive tasks on your list and address them.

Study your list and determine which items are time sensitive and need to be handled, then set a timeline sooner rather than later. Combine your list of dreams and find out which one invokes most passion, interest and desire.

Make a strong decision today to follow this dream because you'd like to do it. Put that dream at the top of your priority list for the next 12 months, then do what is needed to fulfill your dream, plan and pursue a small goal one day at a time for a full year.

Recognize that you have embarked on a new journey-a healthier journey which will bring joy, reward, success and fulfillment. That you raise tension and concern by putting off your goals and obligations. Let go of all the 'excuses' that you have made. You are ready to make mistakes, to learn and let go of them.

You are ready to confront and overcome your fears. You are ready to take on your responsibilities today, not tomorrow. You are ready today to start living your dream, instead of waiting for a better day that never happens. You're ready, do it now!

Each of us has the 'option' strength. We should be mindful of how we have lived and take a deliberate decision to change to new and better habits, to replace bad habits and to make use of all our God-given gifts, abilities and experience in order to achieve, grow, improve and achieve success.

There is no better day for action than today. It is difficult to be flawless, so lower the bar to something fairer and more practical – a high and welcoming challenge can be accomplished and should be accomplished. Just appear and promise to do the best – nothing more, nothing less. Be grateful for 'today,' take advantage of it and make it count!

Recall: I Resolve To Achieve my New Year Resolutions, one day at a time for one year. This is your choice. Do it.

Make your resolution a reality through five basic steps of common sense: Dare to dream, agree, describe, create a strategy and do it every day. Make your resolution a lasting resolution of your lifetime, something positive for you!

CHAPTER 10

THE NEW SCIENCE OF WILLPOWER TO OVERCOME PROCRASTINATION

Procrastination is when someone postpones tasks for as long as they can before they have to deal with them. Procrastination can affect all aspects of your life, such as education, job, time for your family, etc.

It can be difficult, but possible, to overcome procrastination. There are three ways in which procrastination begins. Addressing these areas is a starting point for combating this weakening behavior.

Willpower is necessary to overcome procrastinations, but not enough. Some people feel all it takes is willingness to be productive. However, if you slip and slip, your unwillingness tends to make you feel guilty. Use your willpower to keep you on track, but do not depend on it absolutely.

There are temptations everywhere. You can quickly turn your attention from your work to something more interesting. Temptations are due to a lack of concentration.

The best way to fight is to focus on your tasks for short periods of time, then for a short time do something that interests you. Allowing you to have such pleasures will help you not pin yourself endlessly on them during significant tasks.

Role avoidance is a question that needs to be solved if you want to resolve procrastination. Sometimes we are faced with such large tasks that we are overwhelmed. Because the task is so large, we tend to avoid even starting it, saying that we need more time.

The best way to do this is to break it into smaller, more manageable bits. If you are a procrastinator, don't try to tackle big goals head on. Concentrate on little chunks at a time and soon you'll have diced the whole thing.

Performance in any worthy yet challenging role requires commitment, discipline and tradition. Such elements are central to the resolution of tough circumstances.

Otherwise, dreams may remain as unfulfilled aspirations. Talent and opportunity rarely come together without the inner impetus of the individual. These are similar and interconnected concepts.

Willpower refers to the psychological component that is strongly focused on a mission or a target. Discipline, on the other hand, requires self-control, requiring the real expenditure of time, energy and money.

It is also related to procrastinated gratification or the ability to resist distractions. Habits can refer to any task or behavior that has become a part of an individual's routines.

Willpower is needed to promote self-discipline and sustainable discipline to form good habits such as regular exercise and eating healthy food. Not all behaviors may obviously be regarded as good or successful. Many behaviors need to be removed, such as vices and procrastinations. The removal of these bad habits requires strength of will and discipline.

Routines

Good habits can be developed through repetitions, like bad habits. They usually become habits by integrating activities, behaviors and attitudes into daily routines. Habits don't take too much effort or thought more often than not. They are natural and virtually straightforward that they are almost instinctive.

Bad habits are also much easier to establish because they are enjoyable and addictive. They are also hard to remove. Smoking, for example, is a bad and unhealthy habit that is difficult to eliminate due to the addictive content of nicotine. Every habit of addiction creates physiological and psychological addiction which may interfere with normal cognitive functions.

If willpower and discipline are necessary in order to establish healthy habits, poor habits are also same. Unfortunately, bad habits are often caused by external circumstances such as social or cultural pressure. The poor eating habits of people in highly industrialized countries are an example. Fast-food restaurants serve high-calorie and fat-saturated food almost everywhere in these countries.

Only if there is sufficient reason to do so is it possible to develop willpower and discipline. Extrinsic or intrinsic motivation can be. It can come as an incentive or a threat.

The main incentive to eliminate smoking habits, for example, is improved health either by preventing illness or recovering from existing illnesses such as emphysema and lung cancer.

Will and discipline will enable individuals to take full responsibility for their actions. This helps to achieve success despite problems. Therefore, success is truly worthwhile and valuable when accomplished.

How to Increase Willpower, Become More Self-Disciplined and Be Successful

One of the principles of personal development is to change behavior. If you want to develop, you need to change your behavior to a certain extent. It doesn't automatically reinvent you, but it's still a change.

The whole reason for improving yourself is to improve what you are. Many things don't work for you, because the requisite action is lacking or you just want to make things easier and to do this, you need new skills. Modification of behavior may also mean learning new skills.

If you learn new skills and apply new abilities, with change of behavior, you can take advantage of the new skills.

Our capacity for self-discipline is at the root of changing behavior. This is also known as self-control or voluntary power. You can have the entire world's knowledge. But knowledge is of no use if you do not have the self-discipline to include this knowledge in your own behavior.

You know, for example, that you shouldn't do certain things. But if you still do these things, what does the knowledge mean?

Personal development experts will tell you this: you should set objectives, divide tasks into sub-tasks, prioritize tasks, write newspapers and, despite reverse, have a positive attitude. But if you do not have self-discipline to implement all this advice, you will not succeed! And it can lead you to blame yourself for not following expert advice.

However, what is self-discipline?

It's the everlasting battle between the two. We still have a self that is mindful of long-term objectives.

It gets and remembers what's right for us. Then we have the other self, impulsive and forbearing. This other person is still distracted by the culpable pleasures we shouldn't pursue. This other self is the one that stops us from really taking the initiative.

The impulsive self wants a sweet treat, is lazy and wants to just watch television. Although the better self knows that these are bad things and one really should eat well, exercise and focus on making the phone call and writing the article.

The impulsive self is a primitive self at the deepest level, impulsive, eager, and desirous. The better self is our analytical self. This is the neo-cortex at work. This is the latest part of our brain that has complex functions. This part of the brain has a big picture, weights various options and knows what is right and what is wrong.

Who doesn't want success, good relations, well-being and health?

Who doesn't want to be happy? All this can be done by good self-discipline.

The key reasons why most people are unable to practice self-discipline and enter the impulsive self even after reading books, taking courses and attending seminars; The root of all personal issues is self-discipline failure. The underlying reason people cannot thrive is that they cannot achieve self-discipline.

Self-discipline is the greatest strength of the human being.

You may wonder if self-discipline can be increased. A resounding YES is the answer.

One can definitely increase the willpower he or she has.

However, power is a resource that is limited. In other words, self-discipline becomes weaker. Right after self-discipline, the strength of your will disappears, so you may not be disciplined enough if you have to delay in exercising your willpower.

However, it strengthens if you practice self-discipline over and over. This may sound counterintuitive. We have just said that using up willpower makes it worse, but on the other hand, it is improved over and over.

The best analogy is that of the muscle. The muscle is exhausted and sore right after use. But if you continue to exercise again and again, your muscle strength and tone will increase. If you practice self-discipline purposely, over and over again, you will increase the level of self-discipline.

What are the ways to increase the strength of will?

The last decade of human psychology research has revealed many ways of improving self-discipline or willingness. A psychologist from Stanford, Kelly McGonigal, identifies four ways to increase willpower.

- Get enough sleep.

More sleep is one of the most common ways of improving willpower. In fact, a lack of sleep prevents us from working at our best. When we are deprived of our sleep, our prefrontal cortex does not activate enough, which means that our restraining mind is not at work and we give to our impulses easily.

It's important to sleep well in the night. This takes 7 hours for most people. If you haven't slept for 7 hours and don't feel sleepy, the cortex still doesn't work. That is why it is really important to have 7 hours of sleep.

Meditation is one of the methods that can be used successfully to help you get more and more sleep.

- Forgive yourself.

Typically, we condemn ourselves. We tend to criticize ourselves especially when we have a setback.

Researchers find that, for reasons that we do not completely understand, we prefer to replicate such reversals or indulgent actions when punishing ourselves or when we are rough on ourselves for retrofits.

On the other hand, when you forgive yourself for the failures, it helps to avoid potential reoccurrences.

Learn how to forgive yourself for reverses, mistakes or failures throughout your journey.

- Pay attention to distracting urges.

Knowledge of the desires and impulses is one of the most powerful methods for improving self-control.

It is easier not to react if you can develop a conscious perception of distracting impulses. When you have a distracting impulse or a craving that spoils your goal, you must be aware of it.

We feel various kinds of impulses. You may feel like being stubborn and may refuse to start reading the book or you may feel like delaying the important class registration. When you want to lose weight, you might feel the temptation to eat high calories.

Note the sensation that you get. See and keep track of the thinking that passes through your head. Notice the momentum. Watch the itch. Feel the momentum, what is it? Where's the sensation? Is it somewhere in the body?

Take part in this inner experience. Recognize the feeling and embrace it. Don't try to escape the experience. Face it and accept it.

Take a deep breath and pause once accepted. Give your body an opportunity to slow down and prepare.

Once you have observed the inner experience intimately, bring your attention to your objective. Talk of actions to help you accomplish your goal. In essence, this is your desire or instinct, and then you accept it and continue.

This can be easier for food pulses. It is more difficult to be conscious of your habit of putting things off. But you can improve by practicing.

- Visualize roadblocks.

Generally, people believe you have to envision success in order to succeed. Run by the self-help guru in the mill tells you that you must imagine success and not failure, but thorough research shows that imagining success alone is not enough.

Yes, it's a good idea to imagine success. But a better idea is to imagine failure regularly! You may think that's going to lead you to fail, but that's not what happens in practice.

Two groups of people were compared in one research analysis. One group only visualized the final goals. They visualized the end goal. Another group visualized the final goal and the process of making the journey successful.

They visualized ups and downs of the process, visualized the process and progress made along the way. The group which also visualized the journey was twice as likely to achieve the actual results.

The path to the goal is therefore more important than the goal itself.

What will you inevitably face on the journey?

There are many setbacks and the setbacks would demoralize one with a weak heart and cause him to abandon his target. There won't be only one setback, many of them.

Failure's unavoidable and you prepare for failure to visualize the failure. After you have visualized failure repeatedly along with progress, it is no longer a shock when you are actually struck by failure. You're ready for it already. So, imagine the trip every day and envision a loss.

- Connect with your future self

Normally we don't think much about what would happen to us in the future. We do not visualizing our own future. Our perception of our future selves could seem to be extremely influential in terms of willpower.

If you think that the future self is different from your present self, i.e. if you separate your present self from the future self entirely, then the future person is like a stranger and you wouldn't know much about your future self. In these situations, you don't want to be worried about your future self being a stranger for all practical purposes.

Different people have different perceptions of themselves in the future. Some people think of them as their present selves. Many believe that their future self is very different.

You are more impulsive when you are able to disconnect from the long-term consequences of your choices even if options are not important to potential consequences.

In these situations, you are less aware of your future needs and plans. In reality, we know that we will take care of ourselves in the future. We must save for retirement and we must look after our future by caring for ourselves.

The key is how we can relate more to our future selves?

One interesting tool, used effectively by researchers, is letter writing. Write your present self a letter from your future self or you can write to yourself, note who you are and what happens in your life. Record your struggles today. Then answer your present self from your future self.

The idea is to connect through correspondence with your future self. It is better to be hopeful in the letter to the future than to be cynical. This exercise is not intended to view this process as if you set things for your future self. It's more about feeling that the future self is real, and it will be you.

It's not so much that you'll be the same person now even if you imagine doing worldly things in the future. Like driving to work, shopping, talking or doing housework with friends. Imagine vividly how many years it is going to take.

The overview is here.

Self-discipline is the greatest strength of a human being.

One of the main reasons why people fail is because of the lack of self-discipline.

Willpower should be increased.

Sleep well.

Practice forgiveness.

Cultivate awareness of your distractions and impulses.

Visualize roadblocks and faults.

Practice your potential self-connection.

I hope you can use all these techniques to improve your self-discipline.

CHAPTER 11

ADVICE FOR MAINTAINING FOCUS IN OUR ERA OF CONSTANT DISTRACTIONS

To me, focus means always being aware of your thoughts. Whenever I am aware of my ideas, I am conscious that either I think about nothing, a lot of random thoughts pass through my mind, or just one set of focused thought(s) goes through my mind.

I think that in order to remain sane, you must always be completely focused on your thoughts. By doing so, you will be in a moment or in a mental process where nothing else can bother you. But for many people this is a very difficult thing to do. I'm not yet a Master of it.

It is difficult to stay in this conscious mindset for a long time but I get better and better, and every time I do that, I feel like nothing outside my mind will disturb me, enabling me to do what I want to do really quickly and efficiently.

The longer I do this, the more I can do it. So, I wonder what if in 24 hours a day you can remain focused on your feelings.

But because of human nature, we can influence our thoughts by other emotions and feelings and when we lose consciousness of our thoughts and start to drift into other unproductive thoughts, we lose our focus and come back to a state of weakness and laziness, instead of a move to develop a strong and disciplined thinking.

I have found several ways to avoid this from happening that will help you retain your concentration and use it to the maximum advantage:

Don't permit other emotions, feelings and thoughts

The first thing you have to be aware of is to block anything that can take your focused consciousness down. Consider your consciousness as two walls. Your thoughts are between these two walls. Anything outside these two walls tries to get into your thoughts and overwhelm them.

When you concentrate on a task, whether it is boring or not, if that thinking does not give you a high degree of sensation, it is harder to be aware of it, and as a result other higher feelings can be easily extracted such as those which can be generated by either of the above acts.

If this happens, your initial focused ideas will be replaced completely by other non-productive thoughts. This is the essence of decline or failure to do things when your "walls" are broken.

So, it is not only a good idea to work in a place where you are unable to separate other feelings and thoughts from your focus, but you must consciously block these attempts that come to you subconsciously, each time by building a new and stronger wall.

In the beginning, it will be difficult, but be aware of your every moment to help you keep your focus better. What's happening? What are you thinking?

When you begin to think subconsciously about something that is not what you are supposed to do, do your best to catch yourself instantly. The more aware you are of this habit, the stronger your walls are in blocking temptations and the easier it is for you to work steadily.

Energy Deficit

You are always able to become fully aware of your thoughts and block other feelings, emotions and thoughts if you are at your full energy level. People take their energy status for granted. Energy is like a battery that can be recharged.

Your energy level decreases with every second that passes. When it hits zero, your body can order your mind to close down, making it virtually impossible to suppress all thoughts and ideas, regardless of your discipline.

Your body wants to sleep if you are tired, and your thoughts want to flow freely. To be fully aware of your thoughts is the opposite of dreaming. You want to be in the spectrum where you have the most energy to control your thoughts, not being in the spectrum where you have no energy and where your ideas go loose.

Tiredness pushes you down to this spectrum.

But many people take it for granted, so they don't have anything to do with being energy conscious. A person with full energy would have a big advantage over a person lacking energy, because even if a person with full energy has trouble focusing, he still has the potential to do so, instead of allowing anything physical like fatigue to influence his thinking process.

Make it necessary to get enough energy throughout the day, be it to get enough sleep during the night, hydrate with water and provide nutritious food for your body, because "thinking" depends heavily on "energy awareness."

Focusing on One Thought at a Time

When you learn how to block other thoughts, emotions, and feelings that distract you and have a whole bunch of energy, you must learn how to create what thoughts you currently want to have.

Do this simply by thinking to yourself or about the process.

One example already is the visual image in your mind, such as looking at yourself with a slimmer and fitter body and thinking of approaching someone successfully and talking with a new person.

Another example is focusing on the material that is already presented to you. Like when reading a book, doing mathematical problems or examining documentation.

Then the emphasis is on material formation. This is when your mind is blank, and you are creating a thought. This can be harder for people who lack creative capacity because you start by concentrating on nothing.

The key here is to insert thoughts which can lead you to the desired result and discard ideas which do not. But don't let unproductive ideas and emotions confuse you and overwhelm you. So, first start with a visual image in your head if you have problems with focusing (any thought you want), be aware of this and note it there.

Changing Thoughts at Will

Depending on what you have to do, it is important for you to adjust much of the time in which you have multiple thoughts without any "action" towards fulfilling them. This needs more effort than having thoughts in your mind and while doing a lot of action like dreaming about a sculpted body when stretching and running on a treadmill.

Anything like that would be easier to do than to take an action, like typing or composing, while going through several thoughts over a period of time. It's difficult to get ideas split between your "thinking sheet" or your "two walls" at the same time.

If you were preparing for a math exam, the mental image will split the attention in between getting an A on the exam and the emphasis on the actual exam problems. This is why it is important not only to think, but to change different ideas at will.

Naturally, our brain processes hundreds of thoughts a day. You have to learn to keep what you need and throw away what you don't need quickly. Think of it, like changing the channel using a remote. You can think about it but can switch it quickly, like switching a channel. As you concentrate on your thoughts, be aware of them.

Whenever you think, ask yourself what you think about exactly. Ask yourself if that idea is productive when you answer that question. If not, throw it out. When you concentrate on finding answers, your mind sometimes comes up with no thoughts and that's all right.

As long as you repeat the process of using the thoughts you need when they come up and then discarding the thoughts that you don't need, you will get things done more quickly.

By then, the process basically follows your thoughts with the actions which ought to proceed from your thoughts. When your acts are in line with your thoughts, you not only put emphasis on your thoughts but also emphasize on profitability.

So, ask yourself, are your actions in line with your thoughts?

For example, you plan to check something in an online dictionary, but when you go online, you check your mail immediately. Your thoughts and actions are incongruous, and you can catch yourself while you do so if you are aware of this.

Probably many times a day you do this. I believe that I do. I think I do. That's why you should try to reduce these errors to yourself. The more you can follow your actions with your thoughts, the easier you can work efficiently.

If you are aware of your thoughts, if you are in the moment, and if you follow through, your actions can only flow like water.

Time is Important

When you're really focused on what you have to do, time shouldn't even be part of your thinking. Yeah, time management is important, but it should be your least priority.

People have truly stressful schedules most of the time. They use their entire attention and time fixation. This is only harmful to them because they focus on time rather than anything that needs to be done.

When dealing with concentration, time may be a negative factor.

Too long to finish a task, and you're not even able to focus. Too little time to complete the task, you will focus part of your thoughts instead of the task on time. Time doesn't matter when your thoughts wander away; it just keeps on going.

Don't let the sensations or the thought of time break through both walls; instead, keep being aware of what you need to do.

Allow your mind to rest

Being aware of your thoughts requires a great deal of effort, energy and self-discipline. You may not be able to keep focus for that long when you start. Let your mind stay between your concentrated states longer. It is vital not to strain your brain by constantly being mindful of your thoughts, but to "treat" your brain by taking quick breaks where it can roam freely as you wish.

When you do this long enough, these "breaks" are actually more significant for you.

Most people let their minds rest and roam freely all day long but if this time is minimal, then something as simple as these of thinking breaks must await you throughout the day. You will also look forward to sleeping and dreaming, as this will be your greatest state of rest.

You will then return to your concentrated state of consciousness when you are done letting your mind breathe and relax.

In summary, there are many good mental techniques and focus is among the most important. If you really know your feelings, you cannot only get things done faster and more effectively, but your state of mind is viewed from an entirely different viewpoint.

At first, it is a difficult process, but if you practice it, you will soon know how to be aware of your every thought and to remain sane on anything you want.

How To Keep Focused So You Can Really Start Getting Work Done!

One of the things with which most of us struggle is how to keep focused during the day, so we can really start to work and be successful. Now, because in our lives we have so many things going on, we can't stop thinking about everything.

If you can, imagine that our focus is like a computer. Just imagine the day we try to do our work and we have so many things in our head, like a computer trying to work with 1000 programs that are running.

For instance, you might be worried about the argument you had with a dear man, or you might stress about the work you have to do, thinking about how to walk a dog, or just be excited about something.

What's the outcome?

We can't just focus. So just imagine that your machine has 1000 programs running at once. Is it going to be able to run the software you want to use really efficiently? It's not even going to be able to do that.

The best thing you can do to stay focused and get a job done is to avoid all the other things and all the distracting thoughts in your mind. So, here is a tip and a technique I use to keep focused, so that I can do work:

Okay, you take a piece of paper, a piece of white paper and a pen and you want to take 15-10 minutes out of your day to sit and take everything in your mind and put it in the paper, just clear your head.

So, you could get 15 things, you could get 20 things, you could just get 10 things whatever. You just have to write down everything in your head. So, as I told you, whether you're worried about your disagreements with your wife; you're worried about the rest of the work you have to do; you have to go out to the park, or you have to pick up the kids from school.

All you have to do is write it down, place it on the ledger. The aim is to put everything in the brain, out of the brain and on the page.

It clears your head and can give you a piece of thought and now you've got a list of 15 to 20 to 30 items on a sheet of paper, or even just 10. You must list them to be from the greatest to the least important.

So most importantly, the report you will give your boss or anything like this must be done and less importantly, "I've got to water my tomatoes." Well, it doesn't really matter that much if you don't water these tomatoes, but if you don't finish the paper, trouble might arise.

After you have mentioned them from the most important to the least important, you have to look at the bottom, the least important and simply cross them. You just need to look at them and say, "Okay, I am not going to do so today. I can't do that today. I don't have to do that, so I just don't have to worry about it." Just let it go, just leave it.

So, once you cross the least important things you really do not have to do today, you're going to have a shorter list. Now, the list is a list of everything you can try to tick. You took out all that distracts you, pulled it out of your mind, and put it on a sheet of paper. You can relax much easier.

Once you sit down to do your work, you won't really worry about what you have to do. You can concentrate on the task, the most important things.

How to Conquer Distraction

While time management has a role to play, without your dreams, goals and desires, it will have no lasting advantage. Once you are specific, the results will be fast, and your actions and resources will automatically comply with your desire. Most people are frustrated by conflicting wishes and constant distractions.

Consider these strategies if you want to reduce or remove obstacles in your life:

1. Plan ahead of time.

If it's a big project or a basic call, the effectiveness can be improved with a little preparation. It is easier to concentrate on your day-to-day job if you have both a target and a general overview of your approach.

2. Identify your objectives, projects and tasks.

Objectives differ from projects and projects differ from activities. One of the keys of productive people is to see the big picture, and turn it into a strategy.

The most frequently used process is to distinguish between the objectives and the actions necessary to achieve the objectives. In particular, goals can be achieved by being divided into projects and divided into tasks (or specific physical actions).

3. Set a deadline for this.

You should have a proposed date or time to complete every goal, project and task that you have. If you've got to change it later, that's all right. However, without a due date you will not be able to make a firm commitment to yourself. Without commitment, a goal is just a dream.

4. Keep your goals, projects and activities in mind.

One of the reasons for making the Bubble Planner is to make your previous commitments easier to see. This gives you the courage to be prevent or remove distractions when they appear.

5. Reduce distractions physically.

Think about how distractions are permitted in your home and work. For example, when you receive a new email, does your computer make a sound? If not, why? Why don't you check when you're ready for your email? Because it will dictate your day and your life if you give your environment free access to your attention.

You are on the road to living the life you really want when you are able to reduce or remove the obstacles in your life.

6. Reduce distractions during work

If you work at home or in your office, the majority of people are frustrated all day long. Several different factors, including someone entering your office for a conversation, phone calls or an e-mail, can cause these distractions. Finding ways to decrease and deal with distractions more appropriately can boost your overall productivity.

E-mail is extremely effective and easy to use but can also be one of the greatest wasters in a busy workday for an individual. Constant email surveillance and response as received may seem efficient, but constant small interruptions to your day can reduce your overall speed and efficiency. Alternatively, reserve specific times during the day to read and answer e-mail.

Computer access is a necessity for many employees. Nevertheless, a machine may be a lure to waste time if it is used incorrectly. If you have online access while working, resist the need to search or visit online shops, auction sites or playgrounds during the day.

It may seem like you have just a little break, but by the end of the day these small breaks can be a big waste of time. While you may need social networking sites such as maintaining a Facebook page for your company, make sure you restrict its usage to activities related strictly to business.

Telephone calls can also be distracting and reduce the ability to focus on certain tasks. If you are involved in something requiring your full concentration, allow your voicemail to simply leave a message.

Listen and respond to voicemails later in the day at a scheduled time. In addition, all personal calls during the working day should be avoided, unless there is a critical need.

Training Your Focus To Improve Your Reality

I used to think that focus is a function of pleasure: if I like it, I should concentrate on it. Since I like it, I do some things better than others. Although you enjoy what you do, at least at the beginning, keeping your focus high is not a feature of pleasure. It's a function of will.

Concentration can be trained. It can be improved, shaped as you like. If you handle it properly, it will serve you properly. Today I'll share some of my thoughts on the emphasis and how this method works in your everyday routine the same way you work your muscles.

- Pleasure Detachment

The best way to ensure a continuous flow of focus is to unite with pleasure. It might sound like "rubbish" and completely funny, but it is actually just a way to make your focus more intense.

If you only do things you like constantly, your focus will develop a kind of addiction. It will automatically begin to find nice things and overlook challenging or boring things. This won't throw it off and set it away later, the dull thing actually disappears from the radar. You will end up as a hedonistic prisoner always thinking, "Please just nice things."

Enjoyment doesn't mean you're not going to enjoy what you do. However, detaching from pleasure means you're going to start doing things irrespective of how nice they are. You're only going to do them.

Getting rid of pleasure also means getting rid of boredom. So when you do things, it's just pleasure and boredom. You always do those things, so you can choose how you feel.

- Results Evaluation

Whenever you focus on something for long, take your time to evaluate the results every time. Take the time and compare how you were at the start of the mission and now.

It helps by demonstrating improvement. If you spend longer time solving a problem, you may forget where you started. You begin to circle and fall.

You get caught in a pattern of "I'm not getting anywhere" and your focus begins to weaken. The hedonist part of you will ask for something nice, and you will turn away the problem, for example, taking a cookie.

If your focus is more after the cookie, it will be fine, but your concentration would normally be thinner. You did not evaluate any results, you just tried to avoid a difficult task. Your focus will want the cookie again.

The assessment of results is simple, and it's a matter of saying: "I started this journey 15 minutes ago and I am doing all right, regardless of the fact that I made only one move. You will be forced to sit there until the issue is solved. You have assessed your position; you have recognized the progress you are making.

This works irrespective of the focus time. You may determine the effects of a 15-minute cooking time or a 5-year plan. Holding the attention on both is equally critical.

- One More Step

From my fitness session, I took this habit. Whenever I do pushup or ab exercises, I set a target, let's say 50 abs. When I am nearly at 49, I stretch and hit 50, usually 51, or 52. I've do this all the time.

I did it in business, too. Once I am near the end of a project, I add something else, a feature or an extension. It wasn't in the specs from the beginning, but I felt like I needed it.

Staying in a job, exercise or partnership for "another second" is a great focal point amplification. I always know that after that second, I can do more abs and I always know that after that last feature my project will be a success. I'm in there, I know it, I'm concentrating.

"Another second" is good also for evaluating incorrect paths. Even if you believe it is incorrect, take another second to analyze it and allow your attention to determine.

When the relationship is wrong, just linger for another second to make sure it's safe for you. You will soon be alerted by your emphasis from the start, and you will not have to go through difficult times again.

- Balance your senses

Your focus is on canalizing reality with your senses. Each person concentrates on a particular distribution of these senses. Some are visual, some work best by touching objects, others respond better to voices. Your senses are the gates, and the door opener is your focus.

- Diversity

Try using some sounds in your next working session if you are a visual person. Put some music on, tap the table every now and then. When you do sounds (for example, you are a singer, or you work on the soundtrack of a film) try to combine that with some new lights around you. Adjust your seat, light a candle. It will make you focus better immediately.

In your senses, your focus will always appreciate a new balance. It's not about boredom, we've already talked about that. What you should do is give a complementary signal that helps you concentrate on recomposing the big picture and that will keep it on today's task.

- Your focus is your truth

All right, I cheated a little. I started with all these tips on improving focus and kept the definition of focus out and I did this for a reason. I firmly believe that your focus is actually your reality.

You can't feel anything that is beyond your focus. Everything you do is from concentration, like a handle to control and manage your world and in this way will you live your life actively: if you aren't focused you will push forward, whenever you're focused you will sail.

Now, let's make a short experiment. Look at the wall before you. Take a look. Yes, just like now. I said, do not lie, take a look. Come back here after few seconds and read on.

When you looked at the wall, where was your focus?

Naturally, beyond this book, what a dumb question?

During this period, where was the book? You will say that it was there, right before you, waiting for your return. It's been on your mind. But I'm going to say this chapter was out of your reality.

You may have thought it was there, but it was in a virtual time and space. Your wall filled your real space and time. You focused on the wall and everything else, including your emotions, was overshadowed by the wall. You may have thought you thought about the message, but instead you concentrated on the wall.

Everything works like this in your life. You may think you are doing something, but your real focus is somewhere else. You think you are happy, but you are focusing on useless, shallow thinking instead of real happiness. Instead, you give your mind the benefit of reality to focus on.

You might spend your whole life thinking that you're all right, but you're focused on a wall. You will simply live like a wall, not a happy life. This is why training is much more than a technique of productivity. Focus mastering is at a certain level of mystical endeavor, an abstract, almost hidden art. The person who masters his focus will master his world.

CHAPTER 12

STRATEGIES DESIGNED TO HELP YOU OVERCOME LAZINESS, FREE YOURSELF FROM EXCESSIVE GUILT

Many things in life prevent us from making progress, hindering us from pursuing our goals and dreams. It could be because you feel a lack of confidence, loss of work, not feeling exceptionally fantastic, bored or unmoved to act.

Such feelings distract us from our target and drive us to a corner of despair, faint-heartedness and inaction. There are ways you can increase your energy and overcome laziness when you're sidetracked or concerned, perhaps troubled and agitated.

Here are five ways to do this:

1. Spring out of bed

Start your day with enthusiasm when you wake up. Jump out of your bed, lift your arms into the air and declare, "Today is my day, and I choose to enjoy it." Repeat this statement with the utmost emotional intensity (if possible) for 2 to 5 minutes as you look around your bedroom.

Once done, wash your face and look into the mirror, and give yourself the cheesiest smile you can get from Hollywood and as you leave your house, say that statement again for 2 minutes (if you prefer, loudly or silently), go around your day.

2. Run some errands

You can visit friends or run some errands during your stay and mingle with people like the cashier, or the sales assistant. By going out, and mixing with people out of your home, it doesn't just take you to move and chat, it lifts you away from feeling down.

3. Pump up volume

I'll assume you've got a CD or iPod player and you probably use it on the way to and from work, right? Well, why not use it in a different way. Use this to move, to increase your level of energy and to put you in a happy, improved and active mood.

Listen your favorite music. Start a folder and call it Feel Good Music, then find sufficient tracks to burn on a CD or copying on your iPod or mp3 player. You can pump up your volume as often as possible and as long as you can listen to your choice of relaxing and uplifting music.

4. The strength of images

Cut videos or videos of things and locations that inspire you, make you smile, lift up your mood. Place those pictures where you are most likely to see them, everywhere you go and look at them as much as you can during the day. If the photos are of your objectives, which lead you to inaction, then it is even better.

Look at these pictures as often as you can, even if they take you as little as 2 or 3 seconds, because, when you see them, you will be reminded of them as goals that you want to achieve, that will move you to action, or at least that will inspire you to think of taking action.

5. Daily optimism shot

Have you always felt so weak, unmotivated and too lazy to get out of the sofa before a friend calls you and in seconds you jump off the sofa, pick your car keys and drive to meet your friends with a big smile on your face?

Your feelings and behaviors changed in an instant. One second you felt low and lazy, and the next second you were as inspired as anything.

Make a list of those who you consider as 'motivators.' You can count on 2, 3 or perhaps 4 people to recognize the times when you feel lazy and invite you to take action.

Encourage people who motivate you. Either you call them at certain times during the day or make a commitment to them and especially to call them when you are in that lazy state. Regardless of what you think life throws at you, get out of this lazy habit and get involved. When you fall into the trap of laziness, you suffer the most. Accept the challenge of life and use them to overcome laziness.

Relaxation feels a lot more pleasant and inviting that we don't feel like doing anything. But if we get too relaxed and confident and neglect things, it can have a detrimental impact on our lives because there is a price for laziness.

One thing you can do to stop being lazy is to find a partner in responsibility. It is someone you trust and make a special arrangement with. You tell that person what you want to do, and they'll check with you and ask you: did you do this?

This psychology is simple but effective and we don't want other people to feel bad. This is a strategy aimed at what I call "motivation removal." Since you are emotionally disturbed by having to admit that you did not do it to your accountability partner, you now have a "pain driver."

We humans are driven to escape pain. It is also a positive tactic. You can even improve it by defining certain penalties for failure so often.

For example, you could agree to pay a certain amount of money to a charity if you fail to meet more than 20 percent of your commitments or film a nasty video of yourself, give your accountability partner the file and tell them to post it with your name on YouTube as a title tag if you do not do that. Be adventurous and use something that fits best for you.

On the other hand, the prospect of pleasure is also motivating to us humans. Don't just punish yourself for bad behavior; praise yourself for good behavior. If you fulfill more than 90 percent of your obligations (or whatever your target is), then work with something that makes you feel very good.

This can be a chocolate cake, a massage, a little money to shop, a vacation... Whatever works for you as well. It is best to deposit this money with your accounting partner and tell him to refund it to you only if you complete your tasks.

There are other ways to stop laziness, too-and because all this is happening within your mind, using your mind's power will make it much easier. This is why hypnosis is so strong to overcome laziness.

The Guilt Trap - How to Free Yourself

If people don't know what they have and what others have, they also talk a lot about feeling guilty. When we believe that we have some responsibility for someone else which we have not honored, we feel guilty. Culpability and responsibility are therefore deeply interwoven. Only take another example. Let's take another example.

Even if your partner wants to treat their parents to an early dinner every Sunday. Every Sunday is too much for you, although you like her parents and don't mind doing so occasionally (once a month). But rather than telling your partner, you hold your truth because you think, "This really would hurt her feelings and I do not want to upset her."

First, it is an attempt to manage or control your partner (e.g. to prevent your partner from feeling distressed by retaining the truth). Secondly, it assumes you are responsible for the reactions of your partner.

Perhaps you are right, and your partner is upset when you say that you don't want her parents over every Sunday but that's not your responsibility. Her reactions are her duty. In addition, if you hide your honest truth in an attempt to avoid upsetting her, you will try to manage and control your partner by choosing what you share and do not share.

Know that trying to control your partner by deciding which truths you share and which ones you hide is not fair. Also, please remember that, whatever influence you believe you are gaining; it is simply the illusion of power and control that you share in attempting to control your partner's behavior.

It's not true control and power. The fact is that you are really and truly responsible for none other than yourself (the exception here are your children-up to a certain age / point).

Calling for action

Each of you is responsible in your relationship for how you feel, and each of you has a right to your feelings. Find out how many times a day you think you have responsibility for how your partner feels.

How often are you guilty of expressing your feelings / needs?

It will give you an idea of how much you can control your partner and how much undue burden you might put on your partner.

Something else to try here

If you feel daring enough to share your truth and it is upset, see whether you can do the following:

(1) give room to your partner for his or her feelings (rather than attempting to change his or her feelings);

(2) recognize and empathize with the feelings of your partner; and

(3) stand by your truth, not out of anger or distrust. Just stand by it because it is the truth to you, honestly.

CHAPTER 13

WAYS TO PLAN YOUR WEEK, SO PROCRASTINATION IS NEVER AN OPTION

Planning your week isn't an easy job. It has a lot to do. There's never enough time in the day to do it all. To achieve success, however, you must first address the most important things, then the other things can come after.

The best way to do this is to plan your first week on Monday morning. Check your email, timetable and to-do list. Determine what you have to do for the week. Write down the events in your electronic organizer.

How do you determine the most important things?

Think about your role. As a boss, one of the primary duties is to support those who do the work to improve their service to customers. It is important to take care of the group and to improve its performance.

Yet you're not a martyr; you have to fight for yourself, too. You and your team members need to learn and develop, so make sure that you and your team spend time each week. You still need plenty of time to focus on the other important areas, such as your clients and the administrative tasks of your boss.

Block off time for each task on your schedule.

For each activity, give yourself extra time. For example, if it takes you two hours to plan your budget, allocate three.

Set time aside to prepare for meetings. Why?

Since one of the key reasons for meetings is that the participants don't get packed, don't make that error. Limit your meetings as well. You can't do much if you're in meetings all day long.

Once your schedule has been set, try to honor it very hard. Changes to the schedule should not be the rule but the exception. For example, if anyone calls to arrange a meeting during your week, tell them you can't do it at that time.

Look at your schedule to see if another time is free. When your week is booked, plan it for the following week. Limit chats as well. If anyone chats through your office, ask whether you can continue the discussion later.

Schedule a meeting, if necessary.

Turn off your e-mail chime.

Focus on the task at hand.

If you have free time, after completing your most important items all day, pick something from your to-do list for a future day or a lower priority item. Do the same for the next week.

The following Monday, review your list of things from the last week and cross-check them. Most, if not all of the tasks were ideally completed. Transfer the unfinished activities to the current list for the new week, and then restart the efforts to complete them week.

Make the undertaking more effective methods. Start with organizing your work week. Maybe this Sunday evening or Monday morning. Do it. It may take you more than an hour to complete the first time. It should take half an hour or less if you do it a couple of times. It will be your week's most critical half-hour.

Plan Your Week in Advance And Include Your Spouse/Kids

Managing your home successfully includes spending time nurturing relationships. Let's discuss how you can save time by getting your spouse helping out around the house and planning your week in advance to include your spouse and/or children to spend some of that saved time with.

The easiest way to find the time is to take it from the time you waste.

We will say less about tasks that improve relationships such as laundry, housework, and cooking.

Although these activities may not usually be called "relationship improvement," they can and should be... (besides being building blocks for your children)-double what you do along with those most important things in your life. This is really important because it is something you NEED to do, and you can see from a totally different point of view.

Now, as I speak from the old-fashioned concept of the man who works outside the house and the woman in charge of the house, I have just one thing to say....

The 40's have shrunk.

This is for those of you who have never heard, that the men no longer have to work so hard in the field... which is why we women were totally responsible for cooking and cleaning. Everyone had a place and a job.

Those are GONE days! Men can... and should... help with housework, in the kitchen.

But... just because the times have changed does not mean that the minds of men have changed. Many men were brought up with old-fashioned models... Papa came from work and watched TV.

That's the way it was at my house, I know.

But even if that is the way they act; many men would be glad to help if they knew you only needed it. That is a fact we women still find difficult to express (I am guilty of it).

They would be particularly keen to help if it gave them more time with you.

The key is to plan your week in advance to see when (even) small pieces of time are available. Then proceed to fill up those periods with your wife or child's plans ... because I guarantee you... expected or not... SOMETHING fills the time slot... inclusive if it's just the television.

This way, if you spend time with your spouse, you'll know that you're going to have 2 hours on Thursday night, and you can plan a beach trip or plan a walk by sunset. Meanwhile... he can help you keep things going smoothly during the week to give you free time... and maybe even more.

Your Weekly Schedule

Step 1

Key components of your weekly program

Planning

Work: groups, telephone calls, prospects interviews, etc.

Administration tasks

Auto-development

Relaxation and refreshment.

Even if I don't know you personally, I am confident that you don't like to do at least one of the items in the list and you avoid it. If you start to avoid one of these (perhaps in the measure of avoiding putting it on your calendar!), return to your REASON and remember.

You are in the service of a higher objective. You can't do that by avoiding situations that make you unhappy. On the practical side, you save time by just doing it right away, instead of wasting endless time avoiding the enjoyable activities. You're going to be happier because they're done too. You will also feel more confident about your abilities, because through practice and repetition you will get better and faster at it.

Step 2

Planning is essential

The best way to start the week or end the week is to prepare. You can think about what happened last week, how you want to change your priorities and your timetable and see what's next.

Making sure you concentrate on issues of high importance such as:

What is the most important thing to build my business?

What are the things I can delegate?

What tasks can I do, which are valuable tasks for my company?

Additional questions to answer in your spare time: Am I on track to achieve my objectives? What do I have to do next? When you consider your progress towards your targets, you have to keep up with the numbers, whether you're a "number person" or not.

Personally, I think that seeing you increase your income will turn anyone into a "number person," as the results are so satisfying! Following your progress every week, by numbers or other milestones, will give you plenty of time to adapt your work along the way.

The unexpected happens and sometimes your plan gets thrown out. Keep track of what needs to change in the week or month to come and keep going.

Target big chunks for time planning

Anything that needs focus needs a continuous period of time-one hour is great. Six to 10 minutes bursts won't be as good as a 60-minute burst.

Event

You can still have great inspiration everywhere-this doesn't preclude it.

So, it takes some of your time to determine what happened last week and what things you want to do this week. When you have a list of tasks this week, assign them according to priority. This can be as nuanced or straightforward as you like.

Some people may want to have 3 priority levels: it must be nice, optional, and use colored stylus or a computer program to track it. Others only focus or perform the most important activities of the week.

Step 3

Include relaxation and charging time

This may seem like an odd step for a time management show, but it isn't. The belief that it really is about controlling yourself and your resources is the key behind good time management. You will find out how to keep your energy up and let go of forms that dissipate your energy.

I think of an ideal life as one where I can work with a laser beam emphasis in my company and then go out and relax with equal delight.

What is relaxing and recharging you?

Some people do this by communicating with nature; others by engaging with human beings; others by analyzing themselves. I think a mix of all 3 is good, personally.

Every week, whatever your normal preference is to spend your time, make sure you plan something the opposite. If you are very vigorous and love people, your challenge would be to find some time alone, to do something that you like; for example, reading or puzzling.

Make sure that you plan with friends and family if you're reserved and enjoy spending time alone. This supports you for a while and binds you to your significant relationships.

Calling for action

Include one of these practices on your weekly calendar. It will almost definitely change your results if you change what you spend your time on. This is how we spend our time here and now; it is what really matters. If you are fed up with how you interact with time, change it.

CHAPTER 14

HOW TO BECOME A MASTER OF PROCRASTINATION IN 2020

The New Year offers new opportunities for improvement. In the meantime, you may have already set new targets for 2020. You may strive for a different perspective or approach to achieve a real challenge for the New Year.

My advice is to develop your understanding, whether you are a managing director of your own business or a senior manager in a large corporation, a basic term that must be deeply grasped by you: de-control.

We can all procrastinate to some degree, but could you call yourself perhaps a master later? If not, read on, as I have listed the top ten areas that you can concentrate on this year, if you are committed to this objective.

So how can you upgrade your average performance this year?

Don't forget that if you want to make improvements it must be you who takes action. Make notes as you go through this chapter: what would you do differently?

1. Set UNINSPIRING and DEMOTIVATING goals.

The professional procrastinator cannot be inspired so do not set goals that will improve or encourage you to achieve your life or financial stability. Keep your goals plain and earthly. You will be well on your way to developing your procrastination skills by following this easy first suggestion.

2. Put much TIME into MEETINGS.

An excellent way to waste your time and feel very guilty is to fill your calendar with meetings and become more and more inaccessible. Committee meetings are the best type of meetings for dedicated procrastinators. You also go in circles looking for consensus. For as many of these as possible, volunteer.

Maximize the length of meetings by:

-- making sure they still have comfortable chairs in large spaces.

-- ordering a lot of tea, coffee and cakes.

-- not creating an agenda or having any goals or results.

-- Not specifying a meeting time scale.

3. Do endless INTERNET RESEARCH

With the appropriate emphasis, you can spend most of a working day online looking at goods and services you don't need or need, just don't buy.

Never remember to search for power. It can reduce your choices from 400,000 to 15, reducing the time you spend exploring any possible connection. How long will it take? Not nearly long enough, so avoid it at any cost. Keep vague search terms for goalless, endless fun. Specificity might lead to faster decisions, robbing you of the opportunity to browse without thought.

4. Avoid DECISION MAKING

As Dominic Ashley-Timms says, "Decisions are the stages of development" and should therefore be avoided if you wish to attain perfection in procrastination and poor decisions are perfect for advancement. You know what doesn't work by making mistakes, you should continue forward and to refine your plan. It is best to postpone some decision-making.

5. Take plenty of LONG BREAKS.

This approach can be interpreted in many ways. Smokers have an automatic upper hand, so maybe you can pretend you're a smoker and go out every hour for about 10 minutes. Measurably interrupt your focus by starting at the beginning every time you return to your desk.

Another option is tea and coffee making. Daily trips to the drink machine or the kitchen will boost the strength and popularity of your drinking. Offer to get a drink for everyone. Walk back and forth from office to the canteen and check who has how many sugars.

Alternatively, take 15 minutes to assemble a list or table describing the favorite drink of each person and how exactly they take it. After all, doing a job properly is critical.

6. Discover all of the GOSSIP.

By following this step vigorously, you may be more and more sought after as an acquaintance of all the scandalous things. If people want to find out what happens in a professional or personal life of any colleague, you are their oracle.

It works well for the Ego and wastes hours of the day. You cannot move your fingers on the keyboard from 9 to 5. You can start this phase with a little eavesdropping immediately.

7. Check your EMAIL CONSTANTLY

When they arrive, emails are a godsend to the Master procrastinator. Please leave your current task and attend to your new email each time you hear the ping. The truly dedicated person checks their inboxes regularly, constantly by clicking the buttons Send / Receive. If so you should not manage your inbox effectively under any circumstances by:

-- Setting different email attendance times. Bad procrastinators only check emails twice a day sometimes. In this way, you will never achieve your goal.

-- Deleting your junk mail before you read any of it. Maybe your filters have overlooked something important in a country you've never visited, like that lottery win.

-- Delegation to colleagues for email activities. Take time to build the ideal message yourself for a personal contact. Feel free to repeatedly delete and retype entire sentences.

8. FOCUS ALL MINOR PROBLEMS.

Tackling the unimportant problems is a fantastic way to fill your day without being productive remotely. These are issues that do not affect the end goal and you cannot devote undue time to muddling through them.

Ask yourself, "Is what I do now essential to the success of this business?" If the answer is no, proceed to do it.

Be known in the office as the person who goes over the things that are not important. If you can become an aunt or an uncle of office pain, this will also help you with Step 6. You will focus not only on your very small issues, but also on the minor crises of someone else. A true symbol of mastery.

9. Reorganize your DESK, OFFICE or Applications FILING.

We all know that an untidy desk is an untidy mind, and there is a double gain to that tip. Fall into an unsuccessful loop. Keep a workspace chaotic enough to facilitate continuous reorganization. Instead of working on a script, spend an hour searching for the piles of paper that you have reviewed unsuccessfully: for that reason, only.

Keep every piece of paper on your desk so that you can spend unnecessary time filing and recycling. Schedule your time daily with the shredder, which is sluggish and sometimes jammed because it includes so much material. Whoops. Whoops.

Some of the most effective organizations, which insist that all memos / proposals are less than one side of an A4 paper, are almost completely removed from their offices. They connect with their team in fragments and not by volumes like a study. This approach will not work for your purposes categorically. Be longwinded. Keep the papers under your desk snowed.

CHAPTER 15

MIND TO ELIMINATING PROCRASTINATION FROM WITHIN

Have you ever wanted to do something you really care about but decided to postpone it suddenly, not once, but time and again and then, sometimes, just forgotten?

Well, at one point in life, we did all of it, but if you need your attention to advance a defined goal, then it may be a setback if you don't do that thing within a certain timeframe.

Thought is a very powerful energy and you start creating it immediately if you lead your mind to think about anything. The mind is the underlying factor of all creativity, and the thought that goes before action comes from the mind.

Your mind is constantly bombarded by the energy of thought through the surrounding circumstances, beliefs, friends, interaction with people, etc., and these thoughts are often filtered in accordance with your personal beliefs or preferences, before they are accepted.

If you have a job, at home, a business, or otherwise, postponing things would not only affect your progress, but it could also cause adverse health problems. In a recent study by psychologists at Carlton University in Canada, stress was shown to be often undergone by people who postpone a task.

Five main areas of negative thinking and beliefs that can impede health were isolated in this study:

1) Only in the mood can people work.

2) The task must be given to people who like it.

3) The task must be performed in one go.

4) There is always enough time to do things, so you don't need to worry about it now.

5) Some people think they work better under pressure, so they leave things until the last minute.

Now, as explained above, these five negative beliefs are detrimental to health and once these negative beliefs are installed in the body through repeated patterns of thought, they become tougher habits.

So how do you turn procrastination from within you to suit your cause?

The first thing is to Change your Thoughts Fully and start from the very beginning of thought imagination which is your mind and ask yourself why you are putting things off.

It is not dwelling about the consequences of procrastinating, such as thinking about the job that has not been completed, and the potential health problems related to concern about not having done it, rather, search deeply from within you why you had to put the job off in the first place.

If a task does not really resonate in harmony with you internally, but nonetheless is part of your required duty at work or business purposes for example, then you may think of Different Alternative Ways that you can do it and still feel happy from within.

For example, I knew someone who had a job of sorting general administration for a Training Organization. Most of time, she would sit behind the counter and prepare the letters, envelopes and other duties for the training. She liked the job at first, but then became very irritated by the tedious work over a period of time.

One day she suggested to her boss that as she'd responsible for the Customer Relations duties as well, it would make sense that on occasions she's invited to meet some of the delegates so that she might address some of their questions face-to-face, which would help her personally feel like she is doing her job more efficiently in meeting the customers' needs.

Her employer put this to the test, and the response from delegates was absolutely fantastic. She met them, and then spoke to as many people as possible and answered some of their questions. In addition, she saw the faces of some of the people she had spoken to a number of times, this too gave her some personal gratification.

In doing this, she felt that she had achieved a target that helped her in progressing her job in a different and satisfying way, and which was also beneficial for the Organization.

The same principle can be applied to most things, you just need to think around the particular issue and work out the solution that suits you.

The outcome will make life a lot simpler and remove procrastination about the task at hand.

You may also want to think about gradually testing alternative creative methods for specific tasks over a short time period and then establish a procedure or direction that fits you and is fully in harmony with your wishes. In the meantime, if you have a task in hand, always consider ways to improve your creative mind power at work. This should make it personal and interesting for you.

The other thing is to always think positively of the job you have to perform, so that you think of the eventual result, and how enjoyable it is, rather than pessimistic thinking about the movements of the job. Make it a happy thought, and really see yourself finishing it.

You should envision the results periodically to match you and focusing on your dream can help to remove any negative factors or thoughts that run counter to your strategy.

The use of the mind's "total power" will ultimately lead you to situations and events that will lead you to the result you are seeking. Take a close look at your thoughts and understand that a task can be split into various chunks to help you manage it more effectively.

If the time you spend on a job is unfair, it is best to talk about it with the people or have a discussion with someone who will give you a realistic and honest analysis of this after careful deliberation.

Stay away from seeking advice from people who are negative and who are more likely to disregard your desired goal.

Concentration of your mind to carefully absorb any task and actions necessary to accomplish it will help you start the process of doing it instead of waiting or throwing it aside. If required, you may consider delegating some parts of the task while continuing with the others.

When carrying out any mission, always keep in mind that there may be adjustments and that should be updated accordingly to your plans, the action plan must be sufficiently flexible to accommodate such adjustments.

Remember always that your mind is the beginning of your creative action and as one successful thinker: Paul J. Meyer once said: "Whatever you vividly imagine, it must inevitably happen ardently, trustingly, and enthusiastically."

It is innovation of mind power from within and when you master that will allow you to banish total freedom and energy from any form of oppression, as you work in accordance with your inner creative energy.

CHAPTER 16
THE PROCRASTINATION CURE YOU CAN'T PUT OFF ANY LONGER

There are some bad habits that catch a lot of attention. Look around and you can see a lot of smoking warnings, eating too much, watching TV or drinking too much. But there is one particularly bad tendency that millions of us share, which does not receive a certain amount of attention, which is the habit of procrastinating our main tasks.

It's easy to postpone what we need to finish today until tomorrow. It tends to leave you behind in your work, unfortunately, and to portray you as either inconsiderate by other people, or unable to manage your own life.

Research the individuals who have the most influence in this world, and you will find that they are obviously very timely.

They finish their job in advance and never procrastinate essential tasks and when it comes to where they are supposed to be, they know that it is important to adhere to schedules and timetables to retain control over their time, and they do not stick to their plans (but rather to their schedules).

That's a major contrast, of course, to how most people treat their schedules, but it isn't off. Here are three steps to break your habit of procrastination today...

Move # 1: Consider psychological causes of disorder

There are many explanations why people procrastinate, psychologically speaking, though some of them are the most popular.

First, your subconscious mind can easily relax rather than actively pursue your conscious goals. Staying quiet or going off at the moment is pleasurable and rewarding, while the mental actions of an awkward operation do not allow an immediate reward. Therefore, certain parts of your brain still want to drag you back to bed, sofa, or Twitter if you don't have good habits.

Another reason people tend to procrastinate so much is that they are simply not motivated by their goals. If you're not excited to do something personally, your subconscious will stop you from acting on it. Your analytical brain may know that your boss needs this report by the end of the day, but it doesn't feel urgent for you, so it takes a lot of willingness to move.

Finally, people with low self-esteem tend to be the greatest of all. You might feel frightened of success or you might not deserve it and so they undermine their own efforts by putting it off until the last minute, by missing deadlines and stopping themselves from doing their best.

Step # 2: Face the Head of Issue

Regardless of which of these issues prevent you from appearing on time or from handling important tasks, the best way to overcome procrastination is to tackle the problem with some clear strategies straight away.

The first is just to make it easier to procrastinate things. The person who puts his alarm clock in another room would be a classic example of this.

To shut it off, you have to get out of bed, walk and push a button. At that time, they are much less likely to hit the snooze button and do it again. This is a basic example, but you can possibly remove obstacles in your life by hundreds of ways to do things faster.

You may also let others know you are working to conquer the problem of procrastination. Encourage you to accept that if you're late, or make a pact with them, every time you miss a deadline or put something out, you'll spend a few dollars.

This simple punishment is enough to make you feel accountable and think about your habits.

Step # 3: Picking a New Habit

Do not presume that you will want to stop twitching and change your behavior. Like all habits, procrastination is something profoundly embedded on a personal and emotional level. You may have a few slip-ups, but if you are able to identify the problem and take action to correct it, be confident you can adapt in time.

Procrastination is detrimental to your efficiency, self-confidence and reputation with others. But if you are diligent, appear provisionally, and refuse to put things off when you can finish them immediately, you will be more effective and motivated. Then the thought of not doing anything appears to be strange to you.

You may be the kind of person who has put things off for your entire life, running from one task, meeting, or appointment to another constantly late. Now is the best time to make a difference.

You will be shocked by how much better you know, and how much more seriously people take you when you are the type of person who does not hesitate. Do not put this change off until later.

CHAPTER 17
GET UP AND TAKE ACTION - HOW YOU CAN BECOME A DOER

Imagine a 100-meter isolated path across the desert of Nevada. You and I stand by a car parked next to you. There are two traffic cones on the road with a width of 3 meters. You have been asked to drive the car without going between the cones. A simple examination, isn't it? Let's see how you do that.

Scenario # 1: You're an expert driver.

Result: Obviously, you easily drive the car between them.

Scenario # 2: Never before have you driven.

Result: First, you're going to hesitate. Perhaps, after all, you can try because there is nothing to lose.

Scenario # 3: Never before have you driven. Nonetheless, this time, a greyhound drives by and passengers stop to see what is going on. You've got eyes on you now and you overhear them say-I don't believe he can do it -He will crash-he's a fool to even try, etc.

Result: You would probably not even attempt to feel ashamed and lose face.

Scenario # 4: Identical to # 3. But I hold a gun to your head this time and threaten, if you don't try, to shoot you.

Result: DO IT, in all likelihood!

Scenario # 5: Identical to # 3. But there's no weapon this time and the audience cheers you on. You are encouraged, urged-to take a shot, there's nothing to lose, come on, etc.

Result: You are likely to DO IT!

Scenario # 6: Identical to # 3. You're depressed. However, at the end of the stretch, I put a sack containing $1 million CASH. It's yours if you want to take the chance.

Result: In all likelihood, you'll do it!

I would like you to concentrate on Scenario # 1, # 4, # 5 and # 6. You tried it in these 4 scenarios.

What do you think?

The answer to this question is the common reason why people take action and why others don't -why don't few people start or take up some task, whether it is sport, company or life in general, or not. Two points are to be noted here.

A) In # 1 you took action because the result was assured. You had no doubt about your ability to fail. You had faith in yourself. The most important point is 'CERTAINTY of a desired result.' And how did you get a sense of certainty?

Your expertise in driving a car. Note: information leads to certainty

B) In # 4, although you were not CERTAIN of the outcome, you took action. Why?

Because your environment was encouraging. Your life has helped you grow stronger, improve and try. Since your world has taken care of your success.

Please note: your acts are determined by your surroundings.

C) At # 5, because of the fear of losing your life, you took action. Precisely, it was the concern that MORE would be lost rather than FACE. You had to risk more if you didn't try.

Please note: Fear of losing more than the challenge dictates your actions.

D) You took action in # 6 because the intervention reward was tempting. Of course, you would not take action if you didn't need money and were a hermit. Yet if you were a regular every day guy, you would find a million dollars attractive.

Note: Social BENEFITS affect behavior

In summarize, three factors contribute in fundamental action; A) awareness B) fear of losing C) desire for personal advantage.

How you inspire change in others depends on your personality and life's philosophy. I've chosen 'A.' Some people are doers of creation. Others think about doing something, but never get anything done at the end of the day.

So, how can you go from a "thinker" to a "doer?"

Next, you have to take the right approach. Those who stand up and take action tend to be coordinated very well. You can move from one task to the next without much effort.

Thus, if you always appear to be disorganized, drowning in a flood of papers, or unable to move gears at once, you have to change the way you think. You will be one step closer to taking action once you get organized!

You probably are right, if it seems like "doers" have more energy than you do. Because of being rewarded with more stamina, "doers" will rely on practice. It gives them a surge of adrenaline and therefore an increase in energy!

On the other hand, "thinkers" spend the whole day floundering. So, at the end of the day, nothing was done-but they felt drained! They get distracted and feel much more drained if they try to determine how much progress has been made (or, in their case, HASN'T been made). This is a dangerous cycle! A risky one.

All right, so how do you get out of the cycle?

- Make a to-do list.

In this way. you'll know all you need to do. Better still; prioritize your list so that you know where to start. Then you will feel satisfaction when you cross the items off the list and get the adrenaline rush "doers!"

- Reward yourself.

Give yourself a pat on the back when you scratch off all on your to-do list. This is a great victory, after all! You will be looking forward to these bonuses if you are honest with yourself-and recompense yourself for working hard (not cheating!). They're going to give you a rush of adrenaline that keeps you wanting more!

- Tap into the visualization capacity.

When you have a very critical or challenging mission, close your eyes and imagine how to do it. Once you see yourself doing it, you will have the strength that you need to go out and really do something!

(The details are the biggest key to visualization. So, if you imagine yourself doing something, focus on everything that is "little" from beginning to end!)

- Construct your own adrenaline.

Even a small achievement gives you a rush of adrenaline. Take this energy and use it for the next task. Think of it as a marathon preparation-every kilometer you run will prepare you more for the big race. You will have the energy to get out and take action if you build on these waves of adrenaline!

- Concentrate on solutions.

Their approach to problems is a great difference between "doers" and "thinkers." "Doers" appear to look at the world with an attitude of "can do" – implying they assume that any question has a solution.

"Thinkers" tend to have a mentality of "can't do," which means that certain issues cannot be solved. Regardless of the obstacles you face, clear your mind and concentrate. It might take a while, but you

136

will obtain a solution!

- Find other "doers."

Most content people are the action-takers out there. The more you spend with them, the happier you are. Associating them will help to shift your mindset and ultimately your way of behaving!

CONCLUSION

"Now I feel tired, I will... Tomorrow." Are you familiar with these words? These words are strongly linked to one of the most common (bad) habits in many of us, called procrastination.

Unfortunately, Procrastination is not only a bad habit for some of us, it's our way of life. There are many "occupied" men and women around the world who work all day long and are busy 24-7. But what they didn't know was that they wanted to postpone their vital tasks and duties by concentrating on an endless trivial role in their lives.

People who procrastinate essentially decide to procrastinate their responsibilities and postpone their important tasks indefinitely. Although they can escape the pain of working on those tasks for the short term, all these works will eventually haunt them again and make them even more stressed than ever before.

Procrastinating is a costly practice. We also found that one approach that will not make us slowdown is to find out the dollar sum of something that is not finished due to slacking. When you find yourself in charge of an important task but can feel the lazy spirit in you trying to surface, just say the following three words loud to yourself: "DO IT NOW!"

The reason I say you must say it loudly is because the human mind is conditioned to receive signals, which include both visual and audio signals, from the environment.

By clearly saying "DO IT NOW" you are giving the audio signal to your subconscious mind that now is the time to act and your mind will respond to your message by motivating you and you will immediately be empowered to do any task at hand.

"Before you can start resolving your problem, you must first find out what these problems are." Therefore, you should identify a list of things you are currently doing.

Another powerful way to consider how patterns can be formed to counteract discontinuation is to understand how damaging discontinuation can be. This can be done by listing important objectives that you have not achieved because of procrastination.

Think how good your life would be if you had pursued those goals and achieved them. Once you realize how terrible it can be if you procrastinate, you will get much motivated once and for all to kill this bad habit.

While the previous tip helps you to qualitatively analyze the negative effects of repression, you can further improve this strategy by quantifying the monetary loss incurred by procrastination. To support you, use a calculator or even Excel File.

You can also add a currency interest into the time you wasted. Recall: "Time is money." Each time you want to put off your mission, you throw away your valuable money (time).

Finally, sum up the total loss of dollar value and see how much you're gaining if you haven't done this. Such future incomes will allow you to overcome "procrastination."

Most people do the same thing every day and fail to learn new things. Undeniably the same old, familiar way of doing everything in your life seems much easier to use. But what if there is another route out there that is even more efficient and yet more relaxing, waiting for you to use it? Wouldn't it be so beautiful?

To explore these beautiful approaches, you will need to take a step out of your comfort zone. Open your eyes and venture beyond your area of comfort. You'll soon find that there are several simpler and quicker ways to fix those issues, you don't even need to wait.